QuickStudy®

for

Medical Terminology

BarCharts, Inc.®

Boca Raton, Florida

DISCLAIMER:

This QuickStudy® Booklet is an outline only, and as such, cannot include every aspect of this subject. Use it as a supplement for course work and textbooks. BarCharts, Inc., its writers and editors are not responsible or liable for the use or misuse of the information contained in this booklet.

ISBN 13: 9781423200291

ISBN 10: 1423200292

Publisher:

BarCharts, Inc.

6000 Park of Commerce Boulevard, Suite D

Boca Raton, FL 33487

www.quickstudy.com

Printed in Thailand

Contents

Study Hints

NOTE TO STUDENT:
Use this QuickStudy® booklet to make the most of your studying time. For easier reference, most of the information in this booklet is set in table format.

QuickStudy® examples offer detailed explanations; refer to them often to avoid problems.

> *Examples:*
> ***Pericarditis***
> *peri* = around
> *card* = heart
> *itis* = inflammation
> **Definition:** inflammation around the heart
> ***Oncology***
> *onco* = tumor, mass
> *logy* = study of
> **Definition**: study of tumors

QuickStudy® notes provide need-to-know information; read them carefully to better understand key concepts.

> **NOTES**
> *Some terms have more than one definition. To determine the correct definition in a particular medical word, analyze the other terms in the word.*

Take your learning to the next level with QuickStudy®!

1 The Basics

Foundation of Medical Words

■ Structure

Most medical words are composed of two or more terms. To define a medical word:

- divide the word into its terms
- analyze the terms
- define the word

Examples:

Pericarditis

peri = around

card = heart

itis = inflammation

Definition: inflammation around the heart

Oncology

onco = tumor, mass

logy = study of

Definition: study of tumors

■ Terms

Term + Term (.....+.....) = medical word

There are five categories of terms:

- Prefix: beginning of a word
  (*ex.*, ***pre*____**; ***post*_____**)
  Designated by a "____" after the term
- Suffix: ending of a word
  (*ex.*, _____***stomy***; _____***itis***)
  Designated by a "____" before the term

- Root: foundation/base of a word (*ex.*, ***hepat; gastr***)
- Combining vowel: vowel (usually "o") added to a root (*ex.*, ***gastro)***

  Use a combining vowel when joining:

  > Root to another root (ex., gastrohepatitis)

  > Root to a suffix beginning with a consonant (*ex.*, ***cardiomegaly***)
- Combining form: root + vowel (*ex.*, **hepat/o; gastr/o**)

Designated by a "/" between the root and vowel

Examples:

Hyperleukocytosis

hyper (prefix) = excessive
leuko (combining form) = white
cyt (root) = cell
osis (suffix) = condition of

Definition: condition of excessive white blood cells (leukocytes)

Hematotoxic

hemato (combining form) = blood
tox (root) = poison
ic (suffix) = pertaining to

Definition: pertaining to blood poisoning

NOTES

Some terms have more than one definition. To determine the correct definition in a particular medical word, analyze the other terms in the word.

Example:

Poliomyelitis

polio = gray (matter)
myel = spinal cord, bone marrow
itis = inflammation

Definition: inflammation of the gray matter of the spinal cord. As the note on the previous page explains, you often have to analyze the word's component terms to be able to define it. Bone marrow has no gray matter, so **myel** must refer to the spinal cord in the above example.

- Some terms may function as a root/combining form in one word and a suffix in another word. Classification depends upon the specific medical word.

Examples:

Cytology

cyto (combining form) = cell
logy (suffix) = study of

Definition: study of cells

Erythrocyte

erythro (combining form) = red
cyte (suffix) = cell

Definition: red blood cell

The Human Body – General

■ Development

Cells; tissues; organs; systems; organism

- **Cells:** Major Components
  > Cell membrane
  > Cytoplasm
  > Nucleus

- **Tissues:** Primary Types
  > Connective
  > Epithelium
  > Muscle
  > Nervous
- **Organs**
  > Composed of two or more different tissues
  > Have specific functions
- **Systems:** Related organs with common functions
- **Organism:** A living person

■ Cavities

Spaces containing organs

- **Dorsal**
  > Cranial
  > Vertebral (spinal)
- **Ventral**
  > Abdominal
  > Pelvic
  > Thoracic

■ Planes

Imaginary flat surfaces

- **Frontal** – anterior/posterior
- **Sagittal** – right/left
- **Transverse** – upper/lower

Positions

Reference points for location or direction

- **Anterior/Ventral** – front of the body
  Posterior/Dorsal – back of the body
- **Deep** – away from the surface
  Superficial – on the surface
- **Inferior** – situated below
  Superior – situated above
- **Lateral** – pertaining to the side
- **Medial** – pertaining to the middle
- **Prone** – lying face down
  Supine – lying face up

Terms	Definitions	Words
acid/o	acid, sour, bitter	*acidity*
acu-	needle	*acupuncture*
acu/o, acut/o	sharp, severe	*subacute*
adip/o	fat	*adiponecrosis*
aer/o	air, gas	*aerophagy*
agit/o	rapidity, restlessness	*agitophasia*
-algia	pain	*cephalalgia*
ambul/o	to walk	*ambulatory*
anomal/o	irregular	*anomaly*
anthrac/o	coal, carbon, carbuncle	*anthracosis*
anthrop/o	man, human being	*anthropometry*
antr/o	antrum	*antrotomy*
aphth/o	ulcer	*aphthosis*
apic/o	apex	*apicotomy*
aque/o	water	*aqueous*

atmo-	steam, vapor	*atmometer*
axi/o	axis	*abaxial*
bar/o	weight, pressure	*barotrauma*
bary-	heavy, dull, hard	*baryphonia*
-basia	walking	*brachybasia*
batho-, bathy-	deep, depth	*bathycardia*
bi/o, bio-	life, living	*biogenesis*
blast/o, -blast	early embryonic stage, immature	*blastocyte*
calcul/o, -calculia	to compute	*dyscalculia*
calor/i	heat	*calorimetry*
campt/o	bent	*camptocormia*
caps/o, capsul/o	capsule, container	*capsulitis*
carcin/o	cancer	*carcinolysis*
cari/o	caries, rottenness	*cariogenic*
-cataphasia	affirmation	*acataphasia*
cathar/o, cathart/o	cleansing, purging	*catharsis*
-cathisia, -kathisia	sitting	*acathisia*
caud/o	tail	*caudal*
cav/o, cavit/o	hollow, cavity	*cavitation*
chem/o	chemical, chemistry	*chemosurgery*
chron/o	time, timing	*chronobiology*
clin/o	to slope, bend	*clinocephaly*
-coimesis	sleeping	*dyscoimesis*
-coma	deep sleep	*semicoma*

consci/o	awareness, aware	*unconscious*
constrict/o	narrowing, binding	*vasoconstriction*
contus/o	to bruise	*contusion*
corpor/o	body	*corporeal*
critic/o	crisis, dangerous	*critical*
cry/o	cold	*cryotherapy*
cyt/o, -cyte	cell	*cytocide*
dem/o	people	*epidemic*
desicc/o	to dry	*electrodesiccation*
dilat/o	to enlarge, expand	*vasodilator*
dolich/o	long	*dolichofacial*
dolor/o	pain	*dolorogenic*
dors/o	back	*dorsoventral*
duct/o	to lead	*conduction*
dynam/o	power, strength	*dynamometer*
-dynia	pain	*gastrodynia*
dys-	bad, difficult, painful	*dysphonia*
echin/o	spiny, prickly	*echinocyte*
ectr/o	congenital absence	*ectrogeny*
ele/o	oil	*eleoma*
emmetr/o	the correct measure, proportioned	*emmetropia*
enanti/o	opposite, opposed	*enantiobiosis*
equi-	equality, equal	*equilibrium*
erethism/o	irritation	*erethismic*
eti/o	cause	*etiology*
eu-	good, normal, well	*eubiotics*
-facient	to cause, make happen	*liquefacient*

febr/i	fever	*febriphobia*
fil/i, fil/o, filament/o	thread, threadlike	*filamentous*
-form	specified shape, form	*multiform*
frig/o, frigid/o	cold	*frigorism*
funct/o	performance	*dysfunctional*
gel/o	to freeze, congeal	*gelosis*
gemell/o	twins	*gemellology*
-gen, gen/o	producing, generating	*pathogen*
-genesis	production, formation	*neogenesis*
-genic	produced by, forming	*carcinogenic*
ger/o, geront/o	aged, old age	*geriatrics*
-grade	step	*centigrade*
hapl/o	simple, single	*haploid*
heredo-	heredity	*heredoimmunity*
-hexia	condition	*cachexia*
hist/o	tissue	*histoclastic*
homeo-	likeness, constant, sameness	*homeodynamics*
hydr/o	water, hydrogen	*hydrolysis*
iatr/o	treatment, physician	*iatrogenic*
-ician	specialist	*clinician*
ion/o	ion	*ionophoresis*
ipsi-	same	*ipsilateral*
-ist	specialist	*pharmacist*
-itis	inflammation	*hepatitis*
kary/o	nucleus	*karyorrhexis*
kel/o	tumor, fibrous growth	*keloid*

kraur/o	dry	*kraurosis*
kym/o	waves	*kymography*
-labile	unstable, perishable	*frigolabile*
later/o	side	*bilateral*
ligat/o	binding, tying	*ligature*
lim/o	hunger	*bulimia*
-logist	specialist	*neurologist*
-logy	study of	*cardiology*
-lucent	light-admitting	*radiolucent*
lumin/o	light	*luminescence*
ly/o	to dissolve, loosen	*lyoenzyme*
-malacia	softening	*osteomalacia*
-masesis	mastication, chewing	*dysmasesis*
medi/o	middle	*medial*
medic/o	to heal, healing	*medical*
mer/o	part	*meromicrosomia*
meso-	middle	*mesoderm*
method/o	procedure, technique	*methodology*
-mimesis	imitation, simulation	*pathomimesis*
morph/o	shape, form	*dolichomorphic*
mort/o	death	*mortician*
nom/o	custom, law	*nomotopic*
nomen-	name	*nomenclature*
nos/o	disease	*nosology*
nucle/o	nucleus	*nucleoplasm*
nutri/o, nutrit/o	to nourish	*nutrition*
ole/o	oil	*oleovitamin*
-oma	tumor, mass	*histocytoma*

onc/o	tumor, mass	*oncogenesis*
organ/o	organ	*organomegaly*
palliat/o	to soothe, relieve	*palliative*
pant/o	all, whole	*pantomorphia*
path/o	disease	*pathogenic*
pharmac/o	drugs	*pharmacology*
phyl/o	race, species, type	*phylogenesis*
physi/o	nature	*physiologist*
physic/o	physical, natural	*physicochemical*
phyt/o, -phyte	plant	*phytotoxin*
pin/o	to drink	*pinocytosis*
plan/o	flat, level, wandering	*planocellular*
plant/o	sole of the foot	*plantalgia*
-plasm	formation, growth	*neoplasm*
plex/o	network (nerves or vessels), plexus	*plexectomy*
-poiesis	formation	*cytopoiesis*
posit/o	arrangement, place	*reposition*
prosop/o	face	*prosopospasm*
prote/o	protein	*proteolysis*
psamm/o	sand, sand-like material	*psammomatous*
puls/o, pulsat/o	to beat, beating	*pulsation*
-puncture	to pierce a surface	*venipuncture*
purul/o	pus formation	*purulent*
pyr/o	fire, fever, heat	*pyrogen*
pyret/o	fever	*pyretolysis*
-receptor, -ceptor	receiver	*thermoreceptor*

resuscit/o	to revive	*resuscitation*
reticul/o	net-like	*reticular*
sanit/a	health	*sanitarian*
scirrh/o	hard	*scirrhoma*
somat/o	body	*somatotype*
-some	body	*chromosome*
spectr/o	image, spectrum	*spectrogram*
-stabile	stable, fixed	*thermostabile*
-stasis	standing still, standing	*hemostasis*
-stat	device/instrument for keeping something stationary	*hemostat*
stere/o	solid, three-dimensional	*stereoradiography*
succ/o	juice	*succorrhea*
symptom/o	occurrence	*asymptomatic*
synaps/o, synapt/o	point of contact, to join	*synaptogenesis*
system/o	system	*systematic*
systol/o	contraction	*presystole*
techn/o	skill, art	*technology*
tele/o	perfect, complete	*teleomitosis*
temp/o, tempor/o	period of time, the temples	*tempolabile*
therapeut/o -therapy,	treatment	*therapeutics*
therm/o	heat	*thermometer*
tors/o	twisting, twisted	*sinistrotorsion*

trem/o, tremul/o	shaking, trembling	*tremor*
tri/o	to sort out, sorting	*triage*
tumesc/o, -tumescence	swelling	*detumescen*
typ/o, -type	class, representative form	*somatotype*
ventil/o	to aerate, oxygenate	*ventilation*
ventr/o	belly, front of the body	*ventrolateral*
vers/o, -verse	turn, turning	*cardioversion*
vir/o	virus	*virologist*
viscer/o	internal organs	*visceromegaly*
vit/o, vital/o	life	*vital*
volv/o, volut/o	to roll	*involution*
zyg/o	union, junction	*zygogenesis*

Examples:

Ipsilateral

ipsi = same

lateral = side

Definition: on the same side of the body

Pharmacology

pharmac/o = drugs

logy = study of

Definition: study of drugs

Terminology Sets

■ Directional Terms

ab-	away from
ad-	toward, near
ambi-	around, on both sides, about
amphi-	around, on both sides
ana-	up, backward, against
ante-	before, forward
anter/o	front
anti-	against
apo-	away, separation
cata-	down, under
circum-	around
contra-	against, opposite
dextr/o	right
dia-	through, throughout
dis-	apart, to separate
dist/o	distant
ec-, ecto-	outside, out
en-, endo-	inside, within
epi-	above, over, upon
eso-	within
ex-	out, away from
exo-	outside, outward
extra-	outside
fore-	before, in front
hyper-	above, excessive, beyond
hypo-	under, deficient, below
infra-	below, beneath
inter-	between
intra-	within
juxta-	near
later/o	side
levo-	left

medi/o	middle
meso-	middle
para-	alongside, near, beyond, abnormal
per-	through, throughout
peri-	around, surrounding
post-	after, behind
poster/o	behind, toward the back
pre-	before, in front of
pro-	before
pros/o	forward, anterior
proxim/o	near
re-	back, again
retro-	behind, backward
sinistr/o	left
sub-	under, beneath
super-	above, beyond
supra-	above, beyond
tel/e	distant, end
trans-	across
ultra-	beyond, excess

■ 5 "RRH's"

-rrhage, -rrhagia	excessive flow, profuse fluid discharge
-rrhaphy	suture
-rrhea	flow, discharge
-rrhexis	rupture
-rrhythm/o	rhythm

■ Numerical Values

half	demi- hemi- semi-

one	mono- uni-
one and a half	sesqui-
two	bi- di-
three	tri-
four	quadri- tetra-
five	pent- penta- quinque-
six	hex- hexa- sex-
seven	hepta- sept- septi-
eight	octa- octi-
nine	noni-
ten (10^1)	deca-
hundred (10^2)	hect/o-
thousand (10^3)	kilo-
million (10^6)	mega-
billion (10^9)	giga-
trillion (10^{12})	tera-
quadrillion (10^{15})	peta-
quintillion (10^{18})	exa-
one-tenth (10^{-1})	deci-
one-hundredth (10^{-2})	centi-
one-thousandth (10^{-3})	milli-
one-millionth (10^{-6})	micro-
one-billionth (10^{-9})	nano-
one-trillionth (10^{-12})	pico-
one-quadrillionth (10^{-15})	femto-
one-quintillionth (10^{-18})	atto-

Surgical Procedures

-centesis	surgical puncture of a cavity
-desis	surgical fixation, fusion
-ectomy	surgical removal
-pexy	fixation
-plasty	surgical correction/repair
-rrhaphy	suture
-sect	to cut
-stomy	surgical opening
-tomy	surgical incision
-tripsy	to crush, break

Diagnostic Procedures

aspir/o, aspirat/o	removal
-assay	to examine, analyze
auscult/o, auscultat/o	to listen
echo-	reverberating sound
electr/o	electricity
-gram	written record
-graph	instrument for recording
-graphy	process of recording
-meter	instrument for measuring
-metry	process of measuring
-opsy	to view
palp/o, palpat/o	to touch gently
percuss/o	to tap
radi/o	x-ray, radiation
-scope	instrument for visual examination
-scopy	visual examination
-tome	instrument for cutting

Pathogens

acar/o	mites
arachn/o	spider

bacteri/o	bacteria
-coccus	berry-shaped bacterium
fung/i	fungus, mushroom
-helminth, helminth/o	worm
hirud/i, hirudin/i	leech
ixod/i	ticks
myc/o	fungus
parasit/o	parasite
pedicul/o	louse
scolec/o	worm
verm/i	worm
vir/o	virus

■ Colors

alb/o, albin/o	white
chlor/o	green
cirrh/o	orange-yellow
cyan/o	blue
eosin/o	red, rosy, dawn
erythr/o	red
flav/o	yellow
fusc/o	dark brown
glauc/o	gray, bluish green
jaund/o	yellow
leuk/o	white
lute/o	yellow
melan/o	black
poli/o	gray
purpur/i	purple
rhod/o	red, rosy
rose/o	rosy
rubr/o, rubr/i	red
tephr/o	gray (ashen)
xanth/o	yellow

Examples:
Jaundice

Definition: yellowish pigmentation of the skin and other tissues

Melanoma

Definition: skin tumor containing dark (black) pigment

Synonyms

abdomen	air	all	bile
abdomin/o	aer/o	pan-	bil/i
celi/o	phys/o	pant/o	chol/e
lapar/o	pneum/o		
	pneumon/o		

bladder	blood	body	breast
cyst/o	hem/o	corpor/o	mamm/o
vesic/o	hemat/o	somat/o	mast/o
	sangu/i	-some	
	sanguin/o		

breathe	cecum	chest	childbirth
-pnea	cec/o	pector/o	-para
respir/o	typhl/o	steth/o	-parous
respirat/o		thorac/o	-partum
spir/o			toc/o
			-tocia

cornea of the eye	death	different	disease
corne/o	mort/o	allo-	nos/o
kerat/o	necr/o	hetero-	path/o
	thanat/o		

dry	**ear**	**eardrum**	**eye**
kraur/o xer/o	aur/o auricul/o ot/o	myring/o tympan/o	ocul/o ophthalm/o opt/o
eyelid	**face**	**fat**	**feces**
blephar/o palpebr/o	faci/o op/o prosop/o	adip/o lip/o steat/o pimel/o	corp/o scat/o sterc/o
fever	**first**	**foot**	**hair**
febr/i pyr/o pyret/o	arch/e -arche arch/i primi- prot/o	ped/o pod/o	pil/o trich/o
half	**hearing**	**heart**	**heat**
demi- hemi- semi-	acous/o acoust/o audi/o audit/o -cusis	cardi/o coron/o	calor/i therm/o
huge	**itching**	**kidney**	**lens of the eye**
gigant/o mega- megalo-	prurit/o psor/o	nephr/o ren/o	phac/o phak/o

life	**lip**	**ligament**	**little, small**
bi/o	cheil/o	desm/o	-ole
bio-	chil/o	ligament/o	-ule
vit/o	labi/o	syndesm/o	
viv/i			

lung	**milk**	**mind**	**mouth**
pneum/o	galact/o	ment/o	or/o
pneumon/o	lact/o	-noia	stomat/o
pulmon/o		phren/o	
		psych/o	

mucus	**muscle**	**nail**	**night**
blenn/o	muscul/o	onych/o	noct/i
muc/o	my/o	ungu/o	nyct/o
myx/o	myos/o		

nose	**nucleus**	**oil**	**ovary**
nas/o	kary/o	ele/o	oöphor/o
rhin/o	nucle/o	ole/o	ovari/o

pain	**palate**	**pregnancy**	**pupil**
-algia	palat/o	-cyesis	cor/o
dolor/o	uran/o	gravid/o	pupill/o
-dynia			

rectum	**saliva**	**same**	**skin**
proct/o	ptyal/o	homeo-	cutane/o
rect/o	sial/o	homo-	derm/o
		ipsi-	dermat/o
		tauto-	

sound	**specialist**	**stone**	**straight**
son/o	-ician	lith/o	ithy-
phon/o	-ist	petr/o	orth/o
	-logist		

strength	**sugar**	**sweat**	**swelling**
dynam/o	gluc/o	hidr/o	-edema
sthen/o	glyc/o	sud/o	-tumescence
-sthenia	sacchar/o		tumesc/o

tear	**thick**	**time**	**tongue**
dacry/o	pachy-	chron/o	gloss/o
lacrim/o	pycn/o	temp/o	lingu/o
	pykn/o	tempor/o	

tooth	**tumor/ mass**	**uterus**	**vagina**
dent/i	-oma	hyster/o	colp/o
odont/o		metr/o	vagin/o
		uter/o	

vein	**vertebral/ spinal column**	**vessel**
phleb/o	rachi/o	angi/o
ven/o	spin/o	vas/o
	spondyl/o	

vulva	**water**
episi/o	aque/o
vulv/o	hydr/o

NOTES

Some terms have tricky spelling. Remember that ophthalmic has 2 "h"s.

5 Senses

■ Hearing
acous/o
acoust/o
audi/o
audit/o
-cusis

■ Smell
olfact/o
osm/o
-osmia
osphresi/o
-ophresia

■ Taste
-geusia
gustat/o
gust/o

■ Touch
haph/e
pselaphes/o
tact/o
thigm/o

■ Vision
-opia
-opsia
opt/o

2 The Human Body
Systems in Detail

NOTES

Throughout this chapter, whenever a term has multiple definitions applicable to different systems, the system of the section being covered is listed first.

Blood System

- **Composition**
  - Plasma (55%) – pale, yellow fluid
  - Formed elements (45%) – cells
  - Erythrocytes
  - Leukocytes
    - > Granulocytes (eosinophils, basophils, neutrophils)
    - > Agranulocytes (monocytes, lymphocytes)
  - Thrombocytes (platelets)
- **Blood Groups**
  - ABO Group
    - > Types
      - A
      - B
      - AB
      - O
    - > Determined by antigen(s) on erythrocyte

- Rh Group
  - > Rh+ / Rh-
  - > Presence or absence of Rh antigen on erythrocyte

Blood Clotting (Coagulation)

- Chemical reactions
- Clot prevention
- Clot retraction

Terms	Definitions	Words
agglutin/o	clumping	*agglutinophilic*
anis/o	unequal	*anisonormocytosis*
bas/o, basi/o	base, foundation	*basophil*
coagul/o	coagulation, clotting	*coagulopathy*
-crit	separate	*thrombocytocrit*
-emia	blood condition	*erythremia*
eosin/o	red, rosy, dawn	*eosinopenia*
erythr/o	red	*erythrocytoschisis*
ferr/i, ferr/o	iron	*ferrometer*
gigant/o	huge	*gigantocyte*
-globin	protein	*hemoglobin*
granul/o	granules	*agranulocytosis*
hem/o, hemat/o	blood	*hemocytozoön*
kal/i	potassium	*hyperkalemia*
leuk/o	white	*leukocytotoxin*
myel/o	bone marrow, spinal cord	*myelocytosis*
natr/o	sodium	*hypernatremia*
neutr/o	neutral	*neutropenia*
norm/o	normal, usual	*normochromocyte*
-pheresis	removal	*plateletpheresis*
-phil, -philia	affinity for, tendency toward	*hemophilia*
phor/o, -phore	bearer, processor	*siderophore*
-phoresis	bearing, transmission	*electrophoresis*

phosphat/o	phosphate	*phosphatemia*
poikil/o	variation, irregular	*poikiloblast*
pycn/o, pykn/o	thick, dense	*pyknocyte*
rhod/o	red, rosy	*rhodocyte*
sangu/i, sanguin/o	blood	*sanguiferous*
sapr/o	rotten, decay	*sapremia*
schist/o, -schisis	split, cleft	*schistocyte*
ser/o	serum, serous	*serosanguineous*
sider/o	iron	*sideropenia*
spher/o	round, sphere	*spherocytosis*
strept/o	twisted, curved	*streptococcemia*
thromb/o	clot, thrombus	*thromboelastogram*
-volemia	blood volume	*normovolemia*

Cardiovascular System

Heart

- Four chambers
  - > Two upper (atria)
  - > Two lower (ventricles)
- Wall
  - > Endocardium
  - > Myocardium
  - > Pericardium
- Two partitions
  - > Interatrial septum
  - > Interventricular septum
- Four valves
  - > Atrioventricular
    - Tricuspid
    - Bicuspid (mitral)
  - > Semilunar
    - Pulmonary
    - Aortic

Blood Vessels

- Arteries – arterioles
- Veins – venules
- Capillaries

Circulation

- Pulmonary
- Systemic

Blood Pressure

- Systole (contraction)
- Diastole (relaxation)

Pulse

Rhythmical expansion and contraction of an artery as a result of the heart contraction

Electrical/Conduction

- Components
  - SA node
  - AV node
  - Bundle of His
  - Bundle branches
  - Purkinje fibers
- Measurement
  - EKG/ECG

Terms	Definitions	Words
aneurysm/o	aneurysm	*aneurysmectomy*
angi/o	vessel	*angioblast*
aort/o	aorta	*aortomalacia*
arteri/o	artery	*arteriolith*
arteriol/o	arteriole	*arteriolosclerosis*
ather/o	fatty substance, plaque	*atheroma*

atri/o	atrium	*atrioseptopexy*
brady-	slow	*bradycardia*
cardi/o	heart	*cardioptosis*
cine-	movement	*cineangiograph*
-clysis	irrigation, washing	*venoclysis*
coron/o	heart	*coronary*
embol/o	embolus	*embolectomy*
isch/o	suppress, restrain	*ischemia*
-megaly	enlargement	*atriomegaly*
mi/o	less, smaller	*miocardia*
-motor	movement, motion	*venomotor*
palpit/o, palpitat/o	flutter, throbbing	*palpitation*
phleb/o	vein	*phleborrhexis*
presby-	aging, elderly	*presbycardia*
rhe/o	flow, current, stream	*rheocardiography*
-spasm, -spasm/o	involuntary contraction	*vasospasm*
sphygm/o	pulse	*sphygmoscope*
-sphyxia	pulse	*asphyxia*
sten/o, -stenosis	narrowed, constricted	*aortostenosis*
tachy-	fast	*tachycardia*
tel/e	end, distant	*telecardiography*
tens/o -tension	stretched, strained	*hypertension*
valv/o, valvul/o	valve	*valvulotome*
varic/o	varicose veins	*varicophlebitis*
vas/o	vessel, vas deferens	*vasohypotonic*
vascul/o	blood vessel	*vasculitis*
ven/o	vein	*venography*
ventricul/o	ventricle of the heart or brain	*ventriculogram*
venul/o	venule	*venular*

Endocrine System

Characteristics

- Ductless glands called endocrine glands
- Glands secrete hormones directly into the blood stream
- Hormones affect growth/development, reproduction, metabolism

Endocrine Glands

- Pituitary
  - > Anterior
  - > Posterior
- Thyroid
- Parathyroid
- Adrenal
  - > Medulla
  - > Cortex
- Pancreas
- Testes
- Ovaries
- Pineal
- Thymus

Terms	Definitions	Words
acr/o	extremities	*acrogeria*
aden/o	gland	*adenectopia*
adren/o	adrenal glands	*adrenomegaly*
cortic/o	cortex	*corticoadrenal*
crin/o	secrete, separate	*crinogenic*
hirsut/o	hairy	*hirsutism*
hormon/o	hormone	*hormonopoiesis*

medull/o	medulla, marrow	*medulloadrenal*
myx/o	mucus	*myxedema*
pancreat/o	pancreas	*pancreatitis*
parathyroid/o	parathyroid gland	*parathyroidoma*
phe/o	dusky	*pheochrom-ocytoma*
pineal/o	pineal gland	*pinealopathy*
pituitar/o	pituitary gland	*pituitarism*
thym/o	thymus gland	*thymotoxin*
thyr/o	thyroid gland	*thyrocele*
tox/o, toxic/o	poison	*thyrotoxicosis*
troph/o, -trophy	growth, nourishment	*hypertrophy*

Gastrointestinal System

- **Oral Cavity**
  - Tongue
  - Teeth
  - Hard/soft palate
  - Gums
  - Salivary glands
- **Pharynx**
- **Esophagus**
- **Stomach**
  - Sphincters
  - Fundus
  - Body
  - Pylorus
- **Small Intestine**
  - Duodenum
  - Jejunum
  - Ileum

- **Liver**
  - Right and left lobes
- **Pancreas**
  - Endocrine/exocrine Tissue
- **Large Intestine**
  - Cecum
  - Colon
  - Rectum
  - Anus

Terms	Definitions	Words
abdomin/o	abdomen	*abdomino-centesis*
-agogue	producer, leader	*cholagogue*
-agra	severe pain	*dentagra*
amyl/o	starch	*amylolysis*
an/o	anus	*anorectocolonic*
arsenic/o	arsenic	*arsenicophagy*
atel/o	incomplete, imperfect	*ateloglossia*
bil/i	bile	*biligenesis*
bucc/o	cheek	*buccal*
cec/o	cecum	*cecoileostomy*
celi/o	abdomen	*celiomyositis*
cheil/o, chil/o	lip	*cheiloschisis*
-chesia, -chezia	defecation	*dyschezia*
chol/e	gall, bile	*cholangiostomy*
choledoch/o	common bile duct	*choledocho-lithiasis*
chyl/o	chyle	*chylopoiesis*
col/o	colon	*proctocolectomy*
dent/i	tooth	*dentalgia*
dips/o	thirst	*adipsia*

duoden/o	duodenum	*duodenohepatic*
-emesis	vomiting	*hyperemesis*
enter/o	intestines (small intestines)	*enteroclysis*
esophag/o	esophagus	*esophagocele*
gastr/o	stomach	*dextrogastria*
ge/o	earth, soil	*geophagia*
gingiv/o	gums	*gingivoplasty*
gloss/o	tongue	*glossolalia*
gluc/o	glucose, sugar	*glucokinetic*
glyc/o	glucose, sugar	*glycosialorrhea*
hepat/o	liver	*hepatospleno-megaly*
idi/o	individual, distinct, unknown	*idioglossia*
ile/o	ileum	*ileostomy*
jejun/o	jejunum	*jejunorrhaphy*
lapar/o	abdomen, abdominal wall	*laparoscope*
lingu/o	tongue	*retrolingual*
loph/o	ridge	*lophodont*
odont/o	tooth	*anodontia*
or/o	mouth	*intraoral*
-orexia	appetite	*hyperorexia*
orth/o	straight, normal, correct	*orthodontist*
palat/o	palate	*palatoplegia*
-pepsia	digestion	*dyspepsia*
peritone/o	peritoneum	*peritoneoclysis*
phag/o, -phagia	eating, ingestion	*phagodynamo-meter*
-posia	drinking	*polyposia*
-prandial	meal	*postprandial*
proct/o	rectum, anus	*proctopexy*
ptyal/o	saliva	*ptyalogenic*

pyl/e	portal vein	*pylemphraxis*
pylor/o	pylorus	*pyloroplasty*
pyr/o	heat, fever, fire	*pyrosis*
rect/o	rectum	*rectocele*
sial/o	saliva	*sialolith*
sigmoid/o	sigmoid colon	*sigmoidoscope*
sit/o	food	*sitophobia*
splanchn/o	viscera	*splanchnoptosis*
-stalsis	contraction	*peristalsis*
staphyl/o	uvula, grape-like clusters	*staphylorrhaphy*
stomat/o	mouth	*stomatomalacia*
-tresia	opening, perforation	*proctotresia*
typhl/o	cecum, blindness	*typhlectasis*
uran/o	palate	*uranoschisis*
zym/o	enzyme, ferment	*zymolysis*

NOTES

Typhl/o *here refers to the cecum, showing the importance of using* ***all*** *the terms in a word in order to correctly define it.*

Integumentary System

Skin

- Layers
  - > Epidermis
  - > Dermis/corium
  - > Subcutaneous/hypodermis

Hair

- Components
  - > Shaft
  - > Root
  - > Bulb
- Cycle – growth/resting

Glands

- Sebaceous/oil – sebum
- Sudoriferous/sweat
  - > Apocrine
  - > Eccrine

Nails

- Components
  - > Free edge
  - > Nail body
  - > Nail root

Terms	Definitions	Words
acanth/o	thorny, spiny	*acanthoma*
actin/o	ray, radiation	*actinodermatitis*
brom/o	bromine-containing compound, odor	*bromoderma*
caus/o, cauter/o	burn, burning	*causalgia*
-chroia	skin coloration	*xanthochroia*
chrom/o	color	*chromomycosis*
chrys/o	gold	*chrysiasis*
cutane/o	skin	*subcutaneous*
derm/o, dermat/o	skin	*dermatopathy*
erythem/o	flushed, redness	*erythema*

eschar/o	scab	*escharotomy*
graph/o	writing	*graphesthesia*
hidr/o	sweat	*hyperhidrosis*
ichthy/o	fish	*ichthyosis*
iod/o	iodine	*ododerm*
kerat/o	horny tissue, cornea	*keratolysis*
koil/o	hollow, concave, depressed	*koilonychia*
lepid/o	flakes, scales	*lepidosis*
lepr/o	leprosy	*leproma*
onych/o	nail	*onychomycosis*
pachy-	thick	*pachydermatocele*
papul/o	papule, pimple	*papulopustular*
perspir/o	breathe through	*perspiration*
phyt/o, -phyte	plant	*phytophoto-dematitis*
pil/o	hair	*pilomotor*
prurit/o	itching	*pruritogenic*
pseudo-	false	*pseudochrom-hidrosis*
psor/o	itching	*psoriasis*
py/o	pus	*pyodermatitis*
rhytid/o	wrinkle	*rhytidectomy*
seb/o	sebum	*seborrhea*
steat/o	fat	*steatocryptosis*
sud/o	sweat	*sudokeratosis*
trich/o	hair	*hypertrichosis*
ul/o	scar, scarring	*uloid*
ungu/o	nail	*subungual*
verruc/i	wart	*verrucosis*
xer/o	dry	*xeroderma*

Lymphatic & Immune Systems

■ Lymphatic Function

- Lymph
  - > Clear, watery fluid
  - > Formed from interstitial fluid
- Vessels & Valves
- Organs
  - > Tonsils
    - - Palatine
    - - Pharyngeal
    - - Lingual
  - > Lymph Nodes – concentration of nodes
    - - Inguinal
    - - Axillary
    - - Cervical
  - > Spleen
  - > Thymus

■ Immune Function

- Non-specific response – skin, inflammation, phagocytosis
- Specific response
  - > Acquired immunity
    - - Natural (active/passive)
    - - Artificial (active/passive)
  - > Antibody-mediated immunity
  - > Cell-mediated immunity

Terms	Definitions	Words
adenoid/o	adenoids	*adenoidectomy*
allo-	other, different	*allotoxin*
auto-	self	*autoantitoxin*
axill/o	armpit	*axillary*
-edema	swelling	*lymphedema*
-emphraxis	stoppage, obstruction	*splenemphraxis*
immun/o	protection, immune	*immunogenic*
inguin/o	groin	*inguinodynia*
lien/o	spleen	*lienomalacia*
lymph/o	lymph	*lymphangio-phlebitis*
nod/o	knot	*nodular*
-penia	deficiency	*lymphocytopenia*
peri-	around, surrounding	*perilymphangitis*
-phylaxis	protection	*anaphylaxis*
ple/o	more	*pleocytosis*
sarc/o	flesh	*lymphosarcoma*
-sepsis, septic/o	putrefaction, putrefying	*antisepsis*
splen/o	spleen	*splenectasis*
tetan/o	tetanus	*tetanophilic*
thym/o	thymus gland	*thymectomy*
tonsill/o	tonsils	*tonsillolith*
top/o	particular place or area	*splenectopy*
vaccin/o	vaccine	*vaccinogenous*

Muscular System

Characteristics

- Excitability
- Contractility
- Elasticity
- Extensibility

Types

- Skeletal
    - > Voluntary/striated
    - > Movement
    - > Naming
    - > Attached to the skeleton
- Smooth
    - > Involuntary/nonstriated
    - > Located in walls of hollow organs
- Cardiac
    - > Involuntary/striated
    - > Found in the heart

Terms	Definitions	Words
asthen/o, -asthenia	weakness	*myasthenia*
aux/o	growth, acceleration	*auxotonic*
-chalasia	relaxation	*achalasia*
erg/o	work	*ergometry*
fasci/o	fascia	*fasciodesis*
fibr/o	fiber, fibrous	*fibromyoma*
flect/o, flex/o	bend	*flexor*
ide/o	idea, mental images	*ideomuscular*
kinesi/o, -kinesia, -kinetic	movement	*kinesioneurosis*

lei/o	smooth	*leiomyoma*
ligament/o	ligament	*ligamentopexy*
-lysis	dissolution, breakdown	*myolysis*
muscul/o	muscle	*musculoskeletal*
my/o, myos/o	muscle	*myorrhexis*
pale/o	old	*paleokinetic*
pali-, palin-	recurrence, repetition	*palikinesia*
pyg/o	buttocks	*pygalgia*
rhabd/o	rod	*rhabdoid*
rhabdomy/o	striated/skeletal muscle	*rhabdomyolysis*
rot/o, rotat/o	turn, revolve	*rotator*
-stasis	standing still, standing	*myostasis*
sthen/o, -sthenia	strength	*sthenometry*
-stroma	supporting tissue of an organ	*myostroma*
syndesm/o	ligament, connective tissue	*syndesmectopia*
ten/o	tendon	*tenorrhaphy*
tenont/o	tendon	*tenontography*
therapeut/o, -therapy	treatment	*kinesiotherapy*
ton/o	tone, tension	*myatonia*

Nervous System

■ Cells

- Neuron
  - > Dendrites
  - > Cell body
  - > Axon
- Neuroglia (glial)

Central Nervous System (CNS)

- Brain
  > Cerebrum
  > Cerebellum
  > Brainstem
  > Diencephalon
- Spinal cord
  > Ascending
  > Descending tracts
- Membranes (meninges)
  > Dura mater
  > Arachnoid
  > Pia mater
- Cerebrospinal Fluid (CSF)

Peripheral Nervous System (PNS)

- Cranial nerves (12 pairs)
- Spinal nerves (31 pairs)
- Afferent (sensory) division
  > Sensory receptors
- Efferent (motor) division
  > Somatic nervous system (voluntary)
  > Autonomic nervous system (involuntary)
    - Sympathetic nervous system
    - Parasympathetic nervous system

Terms	Definitions	Words
-algesia, alges/o	pain sensitivity	*analgesia*
astr/o	star, star-shaped	*astrocytoma*
atel/o	incomplete, imperfect	*atelomyelia*

-boulia, **-bulia**	will	*abulia*
cerebell/o	cerebellum	*cerebellospinal*
cerebr/o	cerebrum, brain	*cerebroid*
-crasia	mixture (good or bad), temperament	*eucrasia*
drom/o, -drome	running	*dromotropic*
encephal/o	brain	*encephalomalacia*
esthesi/o, -esthesia	sensation, feeling	*esthesioneurosis*
gangli/o, ganglion/o	ganglion	*gangliocytoma*
gli/o	glue, neuroglia	*gliocyte*
heli/o	sun	*heliophobia*
hydr/o	water, hydrogen	*hydrocephalocele*
hypn/o	sleep	*hypnogenic*
hypothalam/o	hypothalamus	*hypothalamo-hypophysical*
keraun/o	lightning	*keraunoneurosis*
klept/o	theft, stealing	*kleptomania*
-lemma	confining membrane	*epilemma*
-lepsy	seizure	*epilepsy*
-lexia	speech, word	*bradylexia*
log/o, -log, -logue	word, speech, thought	*logorrhea*
-mania	madness, obsessive preoccupation	*hypomania*
medull/o	medulla, marrow	*medulloblast*
mening/o	meninges, membranes	*meningocele*
ment/o	mind	*dementia*
-mnesia	memory	*ecmnesia*

myel/o	spinal cord, bone marrow	*myelocele*
narc/o	numbness, stupor	*narcoanesthesia*
neur/o	nerve	*neurotripsy*
noci-	to cause harm, injury or pain	*nociceptor*
-noia	mind, will	*paranoia*
-paresis	partial paralysis	*hemiparesis*
phaner/o	visible, apparent	*phaneromania*
phob/o, -phobia	fear, aversion	*phobophobia*
phren/o	mind, diaphragm	*tachyphrenia*
picr/o	bitter	*picrotoxin*
pies/i, -piesis, -piez/o	pressure	*piesesthesia*
-plegia	paralysis	*quadriplegia*
poli/o	gray (matter)	*poliomyelitis*
por/o, -pore	opening, passageway	*neuropore*
-praxia	action, activity	*parapraxia*
psych/o	mind	*psychokinesis*
psychr/o	cold	*psychrophobia*
radicul/o	nerve root	*radiculitis*
rhiz/o	root	*rhizotomy*
schiz/o	split, division	*schizophasia*
somn/i, -somnia	sleep	*insomnia*
syring/o	tube, fistula	*syringomyelocele*
tauto-	identical, same	*tautomeral*
tax/o, -taxia	coordination	*dystaxia*
tel/o	end	*telodendron*
tephr/o	gray (ashen)	*tephromyelitis*
thanat/o	death	*thanatomania*
thec/o	sheath	*neurothecitis*
vag/o	vagus nerve	*vagolysis*

Reproductive System – Female

- **Ovaries**
  - Oöcyte development
  - Ovulation
- **Fallopian Tubes/Uterine Tubes**
  - Fertilization
- **Uterus**
  - Wall
    - > Perimetrium
    - > Myometrium
    - > Endometrium
  - Parts
    - > Fundus
    - > Body
    - > Cervix
- **Vagina**
  - Hymen
- **External Genitalia/Vulva**
  - Labia majora/minora
  - Clitoris
  - Bartholin's glands
- **Breasts**
  - Mammary glands
  - Nipple
  - Areola
  - Lactation

Menstrual Cycle

- Phases
- Hormonal interaction
- Cessation

Terms	Definitions	Words
amni/o	amnion	*amnioscopy*
cervic/o	cervix, neck	*cervicovaginitis*
chori/o	chorion	*chorioadenoma*
-clasia, -clasis, -clast	break, breaking	*cranioclasis*
colp/o	vagina	*colporrhaphy*
culd/o	cul-de-sac	*culdoscopy*
-cyesis	pregnancy	*ovariocyesis*
embry/o	embryo	*embryopathy*
episi/o	vulva	*episiostenosis*
fet/o	fetus	*fetography*
galact/o	milk	*galactacrasia*
gravid/o	pregnancy	*gravidocardiac*
-gravida	pregnant woman	*unigravida*
gynec/o	woman, female	*gynecography*
helc/o	ulcer	*helcomenia*
hymen/o	hymen	*hymenitis*
hyster/o	uterus	*panhysterectomy*
lact/o	milk	*lactorrhea*
lecith/o	yolk, ovum	*centrolecithal*
-lipsis	omit, fail	*menolipsis*
mamm/o	breast	*mammography*
mast/o	breast	*mastalgia*
men/o	menses, menstruation	*menorrhagia*
metr/o	uterus	*myometritis*

nat/o	birth	*neonatology*
neo-	new	*neonatal*
nulli-	none	*nulliparity*
o/ö	egg, ovum	*oö genesis*
obstetr/o	midwife	*obstetrician*
omphal/o	navel	*omphalocele*
oöphor/o	ovary	*oöphorohyster-ectomy*
ov/i, ov/o	egg, ovum	*ovicide*
ovari/o	ovary	*ovariocentesis*
-para, -parous	to bear, bring forth	*septipara*
-partum	childbirth, labor	*postpartum*
perine/o	perineum	*colpoperine-oplasty*
per/o	deformed, maimed	*peromelia*
phys/o	air, gas	*physometra*
sacchar/o	sugar	*saccharogalac-torrhea*
salping/o	fallopian tube	*salpingocyesis*
terat/o	monster	*teratogenesis*
thel/o	nipple	*thelorrhagia*
toc/o, -tocia	childbirth, labor	*dystocia*
tub/o	tube	*tuboplasty*
uter/o	uterus	*uterolith*
vagin/o	vagina	*vaginography*
viv/i	life, alive	*viviparous*
vulv/o	vulva	*vulvopathy*

Reproductive System – Male

- **Scrotum**
  - Sac containing the testes
- **Testes**
  - Seminiferous tubules
    - > Spermatozoa
  - Interstitial cells
    - > Testosterone
- **Ducts**
  - Epididymis
  - Vas deferens/ductus deferens
  - Ejaculatory duct
  - Urethra
- **Penis**
  - Erectile tissue
- **Glands**
  - Seminal vesicles
  - Prostate gland
  - Bulbourethral (Cowper's) gland
- **Secretion**
  - Semen
  - Sperm
  - Glandular secretions

Terms	Definitions	Words
andr/o	male	*androgen*
balan/o	glans penis	*balanoblennorrhea*
-cele	hernia, swelling	*hydrocele*

-cide	killing, agent that kills	*spermicide*
crypt/o	hidden, concealed	*cryptorchism*
epididym/o	epididymis	*epididymectomy*
genit/o	reproduction	*genitourinary*
gon/o	genitals, semen	*gonocyte*
gonad/o	gonads	*gonadogenesis*
olig/o	scanty, few, little	*oligospermia*
orch/o, orchi/o, orchid/o	testis	*orchidopexy*
osche/o	scrotum	*oscheoplasty*
phall/o	penis	*phallodynia*
phim/o	muzzle	*paraphimosis*
prostat/o	prostate gland	*prostatocystotomy*
semin/i	semen	*seminiferous*
sperm/o, spermat/o	spermatozoa	*spermatogenesis*
test/o, testicul/o	testis	*testectomy*
vas/o	vas deferens, vessel	*vasovasostomy*
venere/o	sexual intercourse	*venereologist*
vesicul/o	seminal vesicle	*vasovesiculitis*
zo/ö	animal	*azoöspermia*

Respiratory System

Upper Respiratory Tract

- Nose
  - > Nasal cavity
  - > Paranasal sinuses
- Pharynx
  - > Nasopharynx

> Oropharynx

> Laryngopharynx

Lower Respiratory Tract

- Larynx – vocal cords
- Trachea – C-shaped rings of cartilage
- Bronchi
  - > Right/left bronchus
  - > Bronchioles – alveoli
- Lungs
  - > Lobes – right (3) / left (2)
  - > Pleura

Pulmonary Ventilation

- Inspiration/expiration
- Diaphragm

Terms	Definitions	Words
alveol/o	alveolus	*alveolitis*
aspir/o, aspirat/o	inhaling, removal	*aspiration*
blenn/o	mucus	*blennothorax*
brachy-	short	*brachypnea*
bronch/o	bronchus	*bronchorrhagia*
bronchiol/o	bronchiole	*bronchiolectasis*
capn/o, -capnia	carbon dioxide	*hypercapnia*
coni/o	dust	*coniofibrosis*
epiglott/o	epiglottis	*epiglottitis*
lal/o, -lalia	speech, babble	*laliatry*
lampr/o	clear	*lamprophonia*
laryng/o	larynx	*laryngoxerosis*

lept/o	slender, thin, delicate	*leptophonia*
lob/o	lobe	*lobectomy*
mediastin/o	mediastinum	*mediastinoscopy*
mogi-	difficult	*mogiphonia*
nas/o	nose	*nasolabial*
osm/o, -osmia	sense of smell, odor, impulse	*anosmia*
osphresi/o, -osphresia	sense of smell, odor	*osphresiometer*
ox/o, -oxia	oxygen	*hypoxia*
-pagus	conjoined twins	*thoracopagus*
pector/o	chest	*pectoralgia*
phas/o, -phasia	speech	*dysphasia*
phon/o, -phonia	voice, sound	*rhinophonia*
phren/o	diaphragm, mind	*phrenalgia*
pimel/o	fat, fatty	*pimelorthopnea*
pleur/o	pleura	*pleurocholecystitis*
-pnea	breath, breathing	*hyperpnea*
pneum/o	lung, air	*pneumopexy*
pneumon/o	lung, air	*pneumonomycosis*
-ptosis	prolapse, drooping	*laryngoptosis*
-ptysis	spitting	*hemoptysis*
pulmon/o	lung	*pulmonologist*
respir/o, respirat/o	breath, breathing	*respirator*
rhin/o	nose	*rhinolithiasis*
sept/o	partition	*septorhinoplasty*
silic/o	silica, quartz	*silicosis*
sin/o, sinus/o	cavity, sinus	*sinusotomy*
span/o	scanty, scarce	*spanopnea*
spir/o	breath, breathing	*bronchospirometer*
steth/o	chest	*stethoscope*
therm/o	heat	*thermopolypnea*

thorac/o	chest	*thoracoschisis*
trache/o	trachea	*tracheostenosis*
traumat/o	trauma, injury, wound	*traumatopnea*
xen/o	strange, foreign matter	*xenophonia*

Skeletal System

Bones

- Formation – ossification
- Types – long/short/flat/irregular
- Tissues – compact/spongy (cancellous)
- Markings – depressions/openings/projections
- Axial skeleton
  - > Skull
  - > Vertebral column
  - > Thoracic cage
- Appendicular skeleton
  - > Upper extremities
  - > Lower extremities
  - > Pectoral girdle
  - > Pelvic girdle

Joints/Articulations

- Structural classification
  - > Fibrous
  - > Cartilaginous
  - > Synovial
- Functional classification
  - > Synarthroses
  - > Amphiarthroses
  - > Diathroses

NOTES

Don't confuse **ili/o** (ilium = bone in pelvis) *with* **ile/o** (ileum = part of small intestine).

Terms	Definitions	Words
ankyl/o	stiff, crooked, bent	*ankylosis*
arthr/o	joint	*arthrodysplasia*
articul/o	joint	*articulation*
brachi/o	arm	*brachiocephalic*
burs/o	bursa	*bursolith*
calcane/o	heel	*calcaneodynia*
carp/o	wrist	*carpoptosis*
centr/o	center	*centrosclerosis*
cephal/o	head	*cephaledema*
cervic/o	neck, cervix	*cervicofacial*
cheir/o, chir/o	hand	*chiropodalgia*
chondr/o	cartilage	*chondrodystrophy*
cleid/o	clavicle	*cleidorrhexis*
coccyg/o	coccyx	*coccygodynia*
cost/o	rib	*costosternal*
cox/o	hip	*coxarthrosis*
crani/o	skull	*cranioclast*
cubit/o	elbow, forearm	*genucubital*
dactyl/o	digit (finger or toe)	*dactylospasm*
eury-	wide, broad	*eurycephalic*
faci/o	face	*facioplasty*
femor/o	femur	*ischiofemoral*
fibul/o	fibula	*fibulocalcaneal*
geni/o	chin	*genioplasty*
gnath/o	jaw	*gnathoschisis*
gnos/o	knowledge	*acrognosis*
goni/o	angle	*goniometer*
gyr/o	circle, spiral	*gyrospasm*
holo-	entire, complete	*holoarthritis*

humer/o	humerus	*humeroradial*
hypsi-	high	*hypsicephaly*
ili/o	ilium	*iliolumbar*
ischi/o	ischium	*ischiodynia*
ithy-	erect, straight	*ithylordosis*
kyph/o	humpback	*kyphoscoliosis*
lamin/o	lamina	*laminectomy*
lip/o	fat	*lipochondroma*
-listhesis	slipping	*spondylolisthesis*
lord/o	curvature, bending	*lordoscoliosis*
lox/o	oblique, slanting	*loxarthron*
lumb/o	loin	*lumbodynia*
maxill/o	maxilla	*maxillotomy*
mega-, megalo-	large	*megalopodia*
-megaly	enlargement	*dactylomegaly*
mel/o	limb, limbs	*melalgia*
om/o	shoulder	*omodynia*
opisth/o	backward, behind	*opisthognathism*
ostc/o	bone	*osteochondroma*
pan-	all	*panarthritis*
patell/o	patella	*patellofemoral*
ped/o	foot, child	*pedal*
pelv/i	pelvis	*pelvimeter*
perone/o	fibula	*peroneotibial*
petr/o	stone, petrous region of temporal bone	*petromastoid*
phalang/o	phalanges	*phalangitis*
-physis	growth, growing	*diaphysis*
pod/o	foot	*podiatrist*
-porosis	porous, decrease in density	*osteoporosis*
pub/o	pubis	*pubovesical*

rachi/o	spine	*rachioplegia*
sacr/o	sacrum	*sacrocoxalgia*
scapul/o	scapula	*scapulopexy*
scoli/o	crooked, twisted	*sciliorachitic*
skelet/o	skeleton	*skeletogenous*
spin/o	spinal cord, spine	*spinocerebellar*
spondyl/o	vertebrae, spinal cord	*spondylopyosis*
stern/o	sternum	*sternocostal*
synov/o	synovia, synovial membrane	*synovectomy*
tal/o	talus	*talofibular*
tars/o	tarsus, edge of eyelid	*tarsoclasis*
tibi/o	tibia	*tibiotarsal*
vertebr/o	vertebra	*vertebrosternal*
xiph/o	sword-shaped, xiphoid	*xiphocostal*

Special Senses: Eye & Ear

■ Eye

- Layers/tunics
  - > Fibrous
    - - Sclera
    - - Cornea
  - > Vascular
    - - Choroid
    - - Ciliary body
    - - Iris
  - > Nervous
    - - Retina
- Associated structures

    - > Eyebrows
    - > Eyelids
    - > Lacrimal apparatus
    - > Conjunctiva
    - > Eyelashes

- **Ear**
  - External
    - > Auricle
    - > External auditory canal
    - > Tympanic membrane/eardrum
  - Middle
    - > Auditory/eustachian tube
    - > Auditory ossicles
      - - Malleus
      - - Incus
      - - Stapes
  - Inner
    - > Bony labyrinth
    - > Semicircular canals
    - > Vestibule
    - > Cochlea

Terms	Definitions	Words
acous/o	hearing	*acousia*
acoust/o	hearing, sound	*acoustics*
ambly/o	dim, dull	*amblyoscope*
audi/o, audit/o	hearing	*audiometer*
aur/o, auricul/o	ear	*auriculotemporal*
blephar/o	eyelid	*blepharorrhaphy*
cochle/o	cochlea	*cochleitis*
conjunctiv/o	conjunctiva	*conjunctivitis*

cor/o	pupil	*corectasia*
corne/o	cornea	*corneosclera*
-cusis	hearing	*presbycusis*
cycl/o	ciliary body, circular	*cyclodialysis*
dacry/o	tear	*dacryoadenectomy*
dipl/o	double	*diploscope*
hygr/o	moisture	*hygroblepharic*
ir/o, irid/o	iris	*iridemia*
kerat/o	cornea, horny tissue	*keratomalacia*
lacrim/o	tear, lacrimal duct	*lacrimotomy*
logad/o	whites of the eyes	*logadectomy*
myring/o	eardrum	*myringomycosis*
ocul/o	eye	*oculonasal*
ophry/o	eyebrow	*ophryitis*
ophthalm/o	eye	*ophthalmodynia*
-opia, -opsia	vision	*heteropsia*
opt/o	eye, vision	*optometer*
ot/o	ear	*otopyorrhea*
palpebr/o	eyelid	*palpebritis*
phac/o	lens	*phacocele*
phak/o	lens	*phakoma*
phot/o	light	*photophobia*
platy-	broad, flat	*platycoria*
-pterygium	abnormality of the conjunctiva	*pimelopterygium*
pupill/o	pupil	*pupillatonia*
retin/o	retina	*retinotoxic*
scler/o	sclera	*sclerectasia*
scot/o	darkness	*scotopia*
son/o	sound	*sonometer*
staped/o	stapes	*stapedectomy*
stich/o, -stichia	rows	*polystichia*

stigmat/o	mark, point	*astigmatism*
-tropia	to turn	*anatropia*
tympan/o	eardrum (tympanic membrane)	*tympanosclerosis*
uve/o	uvea	*uveoplasty*
vitre/o	glassy, vitreous body	*vitreocapsulitis*

Urinary System

■ Organs

- Kidneys
  - > Cortex
  - > Medulla
  - > Nephron
  - > Collecting duct
  - > Renal pelvis
- Ureters – tubes
- Bladder – trigone
- Urethra – tube

■ Urine

- Formation
  - > Filtration
  - > Reabsorption
  - > Secretion
- Composition
  - > Water
  - > Nitrogenous waste
  - > Salts
  - > Other substances

Terms	Definitions	Words
a-, an-	without, not	*anuria*
albumin/o	albumin	*albuminometer*
ammon/o	ammonium	*ammonuria*
-atresia	closure, occlusion	*urethratresia*
atreto-	closed, lacking an opening	*atretocystia*
azot/o	nitrogen, urea	*azoturia*
calci/o	calcium	*hypocalciuria*
cali/o	calyx	*pyelocaliectasis*
cupr/o	copper	*cupruresis*
cyan/o	blue	*urocyanosis*
cyst/o	bladder, cyst	*cystogram*
-ectasia, -ectasis	dilation, expansion	*nephrectasia*
fusc/o	dark brown	*urofuscohematin*
glomerul/o	glomerulus	*glomerulopathy*
keton/o	ketones	*ketonuria*
lith/o	stone, calculus	*pyelolithotomy*
nephr/o	kidney	*nephrotoxic*
noct/i	night	*noctalbuminuria*
py/o	pus	*pyocalix*
pyel/o	renal pelvis	*pyelophlebitis*
ren/o	kidney	*renogastric*
ur/o	urine	*uroerythrin*
-uresis	urination	*diuresis*
ureter/o	ureter	*ureterocolostomy*
urethr/o	urethra	*urethrorrhagia*
-uria	urine condition	*pyuria*
uric/o	uric acid	*uricosuria*
urin/o	urine	*urinalysis*
vesic/o	urinary bladder	*vesicoclysis*

3 Abbreviations & Acronyms

Overview

■ Purpose

As there are thousands of medical abbreviations and acronyms, the purpose of this chapter is to present those most commonly used. **Care** must be exercised when using this shorthand communication format, because of multiple meanings for a particular abbreviation or acronym. The correct definition is determined by the context of the material.

■ Definitions

Abbreviation: A shortened form of a word or phrase: tid = three times a day

Acronym: Word formed from the initial letters in a phrase: WHO = World Health Organization

NOTES

Some abbreviations and acronyms may appear:

- *In lower or upper case lettering*
- *With or without periods*

Weights & Measurements

C	Celsius, centigrade
cc	cubic centimeter
Ci, c	Curie
cm	centimeter
dB	decibel
dl	deciliter
dr	dram
F	Fahrenheit
fl dr	fluid dram
Fl, fld	fluid
fl oz	fluid ounce
g, gm	gram
Hz	hertz
IU	International Unit
kg	kilogram
km	kilometer
L, l	liter
L/min	liters per minute
lb.	pound
M	molar, thousand, meter
m	meter
mcg, μg	microgram
mCi, mc	millicurie
mEq	milliequivalent
mEq/L	milliequivalent per liter
mg, mgm	milligram
ml, mL	milliliter
mm	millimeter
mmHg	millimeters of mercury
mol wt, MW, MWt	molecular weight
mμ	millimicron

oz.	ounce
ppm	parts per million
pt	pint
rad	radiation absorbed dose
rev/min, rpm	revolutions per minute
SI	International System of Units
U	unit
μ, mu	micron
V	volt
vol %	volume percent
v/v	volume per volume
W	watt
w/v	weight per volume

Pharmacology

■ Pharmaceuticals (Drugs)

ACD	anticonvulsant drug
ADR	adverse drug reaction
ASA	acetylsalicylic acid (aspirin)
CD	curative dose
D, dos	dose, dosage
DAW	dispense as written
DAWN	Drug Abuse Warning Network
DIG	digitalis
DSB	drug-seeking behavior
IND	investigational new drug
INH	isoniazid (TB drug)
LD	lethal dose
MAOI	monoamine oxidase inhibitor
MAR	medication administration record
meds	medications, medicines
NSAID	non-steroidal anti-inflammatory drug

OD	(drug) overdose
OTC	over the counter
PCA	patient-controlled analgesia
PCN, PNC	penicillin
Rx	prescription, drug, medication
sig	label
TDM	therapeutic drug monitoring

■ Formulations

aer	aerosol
aq	water, aqueous
bol, pil	pill
cap	capsule
comp	compound
dil, dilut	dilute
elix, el	elixir
ext	extract
fld, FL	fluid
garg	a gargle
gtt, gt	drops, drop
linim	liniment
liq	liquid
lot	lotion
M	mixture, mix
pulv	powder (pulvule)
sol, soln	solution
solv	dissolve
spt	spirit
supp	suppository
susp	suspension
syr	syrup
tab	tablet
tinct	tincture
ung	ointment

■ Administration: Directions

a	before
āā	of each
ac	before meals
ad lib.	freely, as desired
admov	apply
AM	before noon
atc	around the clock
bib	drink
bid	twice a day
c̄	with
d	day
dc, D/C	discontinue
h	hour
hs	at bedtime
npo	nothing by mouth
od	every day, daily
p̄, p	after
pc	after meals
PM	afternoon, evening
prn	as required/needed
q	every
qd	every day
qh	every hour
qid	four times a day
ql	as much as desired
qm	every morning
qn	every night
qod	every other day
qoh	every other hour
qon	every other night
qp	as much as desired
qpm, qn	every night/evening
qs	quantity sufficient

s̄	without
semih	half an hour
sos	if necessary
s̄ s̄, ss, s̄̇ s̄̇	half
tid	three times a day
tin	three times a night
ut dict	as directed

■ Administration: Routes

hypo	hypodermic (injection)
IC, ICAV	intracavitary
ID	intradermal
IM	intramuscular
inhal	inhalation
inj, inject	injection
IT, i-thec	intrathecal
IV	intravenous
IVP	intravenous push
IVPB	intravenous piggyback
MDI	metered dose inhaler
pr	through rectum, per rectum
parent, P	parenteral
po	orally
SL, subl	sublingual
SQ, SC, subq, subcu	subcutaneous
TDD	transdermal drug delivery
top	topically

■ References

NDC	National Drug Code
NF	National Formulary
PDR	Physicians' Desk Reference

■ Standards & Regulations

DEA	Drug Enforcement Agency
FDA	Food & Drug Administration
USP	United States Pharmacopeia

Diagnostic Testing

ac phos, ACP	acid phosphatase
AFP	alpha fetoprotein
A/G	albumin-globulin ratio
alk phos, ALP	alkaline phosphatase
ALT	alanine aminotransferase (SGPT)
ANA	antinuclear antibodies
APTT, aPTT	activated partial thromboplastin time
ASO, ASL-O	antistreptolysin-O
AST	aspartate aminotransferase (SGOT)
BT	bleeding time
BUN	blood urea nitrogen
Ca	calcium
CAT, CT	computed axial tomography
CBC	complete blood count
CEA	carcinoembryonic antigen
Chol	cholesterol
Cl	chloride
CPK	creatine phosphokinase
creat	creatinine
CRP	C-reactive protein
CXR	chest x-ray
DEXA	dual energy x-ray absorptiometry
diff	differential (blood count)
DR	diagnostic radiography
DSA	digital subtraction angiography

ECG, EKG	electrocardiogram
ECHO	echocardiography
EEG	electroencephalogram
ESR, sed rate	erythrocyte sedimentation rate
FBS	fasting blood sugar
GTT	glucose tolerance test
HCT, crit	hematocrit
HDI	high-definition imaging
HDL	high-density lipoprotein
Hgb	hemoglobin
K	potassium
LDH	lactate dehydrogenase
LDL	low-density lipoprotein
lytes	electrolytes
MCH	mean corpuscular hemoglobin
MCHC	mean corpuscular hemoglobin concentration
MCV	mean corpuscular volume
MRI	magnetic resonance imaging
MUGA	multiple-gated acquisition scanning
Na	sodium
PCV	packed cell volume
PET	positron emission tomography
PFT	pulmonary function test
pH	hydrogen ion concentration
plats, PLT	platelets
PT, pro. time	prothrombin time
PTT	partial thromboplastin time
RAIU, RIU	radioactive iodine uptake
RAST	radioallergosorbent test
RBC	red blood cell, red blood count
RDW	red (cell) distribution width
RIA	radioimmunoassay
RIFA	radioimmunofluorescence assay
SMA	sequential multiple analysis (clinical chemistry)

SPECT	single photon emission computed tomography
sp gr, SG	specific gravity
T&C	type and crossmatch
TFT	thyroid function test
trig	triglycerides
TT	thrombin time
UA, U/A	urinalysis
U/S, US	ultrasound
VLDL	very low density lipoprotein
WBC	white blood cell, white blood count
XR	x-ray

Professional Designations

ARNP	Advanced Registered Nurse Practitioner
ATR-BC	Registered Art Therapist-Board Certified
CCT	Certified Cardiographic Technician
CDA	Certified Dental Assistant
CDT	Certified Dental Technician
CMA	Certified Medical Assistant
CNMT	Certified Nuclear Medicine Technologist
CO	Certified Orthotist
COMT	Certified Ophthalmic Medical Technologist
COT	Certified Ophthalmic Technician
COTA	Certified Occupational Therapy Assistant
CP	Certified Prosthetist
CPhT	Certified Pharmacy Technician
CPO	Certified Prosthetist & Orthotist

CRC	Certified Rehabilitation Counselor
CRT	Certified Respiratory Therapist
CST	Certified Surgical Technologist
CT (ASCP)	Cytotechnologist (American Society of Clinical Pathologists)
CTRS	Certified Therapeutic Recreation Specialist
DC	Doctor of Chiropractic
DDS	Doctor of Dental Surgery
DMD	Doctor of Dental Medicine
DO	Doctor of Osteopathy
DPM	Doctor of Podiatric Medicine
DTR	Dietetic Technician, Registered
EMT	Emergency Medical Technician
EMT-P	Emergency Medical Technician-Paramedic
HT (ASCP)	Histologic Technician (American Society of Clinical Pathologists)
HTL (ASCP)	Histotechnologist (American Society of Clinical Pathologists)
LCSW	Licensed Clinical Social Worker
LMHC	Licensed Mental Health Counselor
LPN	Licensed Practical Nurse
LVN	Licensed Vocational Nurse
MD	Doctor of Medicine
MLT (ASCP)	Medical Laboratory Technician (American Society of Clinical Pathologists)
MT (ASCP)	Medical Technologist (American Society of Clinical Pathologists)
MT-BC	Music Therapist-Board Certified
NA	Nursing Assistant
OD	Doctor of Optometry
OTR	Occupational Therapist, Registered
PA-C	Physician Assistant-Certified

PT	Physical Therapist
PTA	Physical Therapist Assistant
RCIS	Registered Cardiovascular Invasive Specialist
RCS	Registered Cardiac Sonographer
RD	Registered Dietician
RDH	Registered Dental Hygienist
RDMS	Registered Diagnostic Medical Sonographer
RHIA	Registered Health Information Administrator
RN	Registered Nurse
R.Ph.	Registered Pharmacist
RRT	Registered Respiratory Therapist
RT (N)	Radiologic Technologist (Nuclear Medicine)
RT (R)	Radiologic Technologist (Radiographer)
RT (T)	Radiologic Technologist (Radiation Therapist)
RVS	Registered Vascular Specialist
SCT (ASCP)	Specialized Cytotechnologist (American Society of Clinical Pathologists)

Managed Care

ASO	administrative services only
cap	capitation (reimbursement)
CM	case management/manager
COB	Coordination of Benefits
COBRA	Consolidated Omnibus Budget Reconciliation Act (1985)

COC	Certificate of Coverage
co-pay	copayment
DUR	drug usage/utilization review
EOB	Explanation of Benefits
EPO	Exclusive Provider Organization
ERISA	Employee Retirement Income Security Act (1974)
FFS	Fee-for-Service (reimbursement)
HEDIS	Health Employer Data & Information Set
HI	health insurance
HIPAA	Health Insurance Portability & Accountability Act (1996)
HMO	Health Maintenance Organization
IPA	Independent Practice Association
MCO	Managed Care Organization
MCP	managed care plan
MIP	Managed Indemnity Program/Plan
MSP	Medicare Secondary Payor
NCQA	National Committee for Quality Assurance
PBM	Pharmacy Benefit Manager
PCP	Primary Care Provider, Primary Care Physician
PHO	Physician – Hospital Organization
PMPM	per member per month (capitation)
POS	Point of Service
PPO	Preferred Provider Organization
PPS	Prospective Payment System
SSO	second surgical opinion
TPA	Third Party Administrator
UCR	usual, customary and reasonable (fees)
UR	Utilization Review

Agencies & Organizations

AHA	American Hospital Association
AMA	American Medical Association
CAAHEP	Commission on Accreditation of Allied Health Education Programs
CDC	Centers for Disease Control
CMS	Centers for Medicare and Medicaid Services
FDA	Food & Drug Administration
HHA	Home Health Agency
IOM	Institute of Medicine
JCAHO	Joint Commission on Accreditation of Healthcare Organizations
NCI	National Cancer Institute
NHC	National Health Council
NIH	National Institutes of Health
NLN	National League for Nursing
NORD	National Organization for Rare Disorders
UNOS	United Network for Organ Sharing
USDHHS	U.S. Department of Health/ Human Services
USPHS	U.S. Public Health Service
VNA	Visiting Nurse Association
WHO	World Health Organization

Health Assessment

abn, abnorm	abnormal
amb	ambulatory
A&O x 4	alert and oriented to person, place, time and date
A/O, A&O	alert and oriented
A&P	auscultation and palpation, auscultation and percussion

Asx, ASX	asymptomatic
ausc, auscul	auscultation
A&W	alive and well
BP	blood pressure
CA	chronological age
C&A	conscious and alert
CC, c/o	chief complaint, complains of
DOB, D/B	date of birth
DU	diagnosis undetermined
Dx, diag	diagnosis
Ex, exam	examination
F	female
FH, FHx	family history
FOD	free of disease
F/U, FU	follow-up
FUO	fever of unknown origin
h/o	history of
H&P	history and physical
Ht, h	height
Hx, H	history
IBW	ideal body weight
IPPA	inspection, palpation, percussion, auscultation
IQ	intelligence quotient
L&W	living and well
LWD	living with disease
M	male
MA	mental age
MHx, MH	medical history
NAD	no appreciable disease, no apparent distress/disease, nothing abnormal detected
N/C, NC	no complaints
ND	not diagnosed
NDF	no disease found

NED	no evidence of disease
NKA	no known allergies
NKDA	no known drug allergies
norm	normal
NVS	neurological vital signs
NYD	not yet diagnosed
P	pulse
P&A, P/A	percussion and auscultation
palp	palpation
PE, PEx, PX	physical examination
PH	poor health
PH, Px, PHx	past history
PI	present illness
PMH, PMHx	past medical history
PMI	past medical illness
PPHx	previous psychiatric history
prog, progn, Px	prognosis
Pt	patient
R	respiration
R/O, RO	rule out
ROS	review of systems
RVC	responds to verbal commands
SOAP	subjective, objective, assessment, plan (problem-oriented record)
SOI	severity of illness
SONP	soft organs not palpable
S/S	signs and symptoms
Sx	symptoms, signs
T	temperature
TPR	temperature, pulse and respiration
Tx, treat, tr	treatment
UCHD, UCD	usual childhood diseases
U/O, UO	under observation
VS, v/s	vital signs
WDWN	well developed, well nourished

WNL	within normal limits
wt	weight
X&D	examination and diagnosis
y, yr	year
y/o	years old
YOB	year of birth

Specialized Areas & Facilities

ACC	Ambulatory Care Center
ALF	Assisted Living Facility
BB, BLBK	Blood Bank
BU	Burn Unit
CCRC	Continuous Care Retirement Community
CCU	Coronary Care Unit, Critical Care Unit
DR	Delivery Room
ECF	Extended Care Facility
ED	Emergency Department
ER	Emergency Room
ETU	Emergency Trauma Unit, Emergency Treatment Unit
HDU	Hemodialysis Unit
ICF	Intermediate Care Facility
ICU	Intensive Care Unit, Intermediate Care Unit
Lab	Laboratory
LR	Labor Room
MHC	Mental Health Center
MICU	Medical Intensive Care Unit
MRD	Medical Records Department
NICU	Neonatal Intensive Care Unit

OPC	Outpatient Clinic
OPD	Outpatient Department
OPS	Outpatient Surgery, Outpatient Service
OR	Operating Room
OT	Occupational Therapy
PCC	Poison Control Center
PCU	Progressive Care Unit
Peds	Pediatrics
Pharm	Pharmacy
PICU	Pediatric Intensive Care Unit
PT	Physical Therapy
RPCH	Rural Primary Care Hospital
RR	Recovery Room
SICU	Surgical Intensive Care Unit
SNF	Skilled Nursing Facility
TC	Therapeutic Community, Trauma Center

Locations & Directions

AAL	anterior axillary line
A&D	ascending and descending
AE	above the elbow
AK	above the knee
ant.	anterior
AP	anteroposterior
A&P	anterior and posterior
BE	below the elbow
bilat	bilateral
BK	below the knee
ext	exterior, external
ICS, IS	intercostal space

inf	inferior
int	interior, internal
L	left
LAD	left anterior descending
LAO	left anterior oblique
Lat, L	lateral
LE	lower extremity
LLE	left lower extremity
LLL	left lower lobe (lung)
LLQ	left lower quadrant
LPO	left posterior oblique
L&R	left and right
L-R	left to right
LRT	lower respiratory tract
L&U	lower and upper
LUE	left upper extremity
LUL	left upper lobe (lung)
LUQ	left upper quadrant
MCL	midclavicular line
ML	midline
MSL	midsternal line
PA, P-A	posteroanterior
post.	posterior
prox.	proximal
R	right
RAD	right anterior descending
RAO	right anterior oblique
R/L, R-L	right to left
RLE	right lower extremity
RLL	right lower lobe (lung)
RLQ	right lower quadrant
RML	right middle lobe (lung), right mediolateral
RPO	right posterior oblique
RUE	right upper extremity

RUL	right upper lobe (lung)
RUQ	right upper quadrant
sup	superior
U/L, U&L	upper and lower
UE	upper extremity
URT	upper respiratory tract

NOTES

*The abbreviations and acronyms from here to the end of this chapter refer to the body systems detailed in chapter 2. Certain abbreviations apply to more than one system (i.e., **MS**).*

Examples:

MS

Cardiovascular = mitral stenosis

Muscular = musculoskeletal or muscle strength

Nervous = multiple sclerosis

Body Systems

■ Blood System

ABMT	autologous bone marrow transplant
ABO	blood groups
AC	anticoagulant
ACT	anticoagulant therapy
agg, aggl	agglutination
AHF	antihemophilic factor
AIHA	autoimmune hemolytic anemia
ALL	acute lymphocytic leukemia
AML	acute myelogenous leukemia

APA	antipernicious anemia (factor)
AUL	acute undifferentiated leukemia
B, bl, bld	blood
baso	basophil
bl	bleeding
BMB	bone-marrow biopsy
BMT	bone-marrow transplant
CBC	complete blood count
CLL	chronic lymphocytic leukemia
CML	chronic myelogenous leukemia
coag	coagulation
DIC	disseminated intravascular coagulation
eos, eosins	eosinophil
EPO	erythropoietin
IF	intrinsic factor
ITP	idiopathic thrombocytopenia purpura
LIF	leukemia inhibitory factor
lymphs	lymphocytes
mono	monocyte
PAF	platelet activating factor
plats, PLT	platelet
PMN, polys, segs	polymorphonuclear neutrophils
PNH	paroxysmal nocturnal hemoglobinuria
PV	polycythemia vera
RBC	red blood cell, red blood cell count
retic	reticulocyte
Rh	Rhesus blood factor
SCT	sickle cell trait
T&C	type and crossmatch
TTP	thrombotic thrombocytopenia purpura
WBC	white blood cell, white blood count

■ Cardiovascular System

ABP	arterial blood pressure
ACLS	advanced cardiac life support
AED	automated external defibrillator
AF, Afib, at fib	atrial fibrillation
AIVR	accelerated idioventricular rhythm
AMI	acute myocardial infarction
ang	angiogram
Ao	aorta
AR	aortic regurgitation
AS	aortic stenosis, arteriosclerosis
ASCVD	arteriosclerotic cardiovascular disease
ASD	atrial septal defect
ASHD	arteriosclerotic heart disease
AV, A-V	atrioventricular, arteriovenous
AVB	atrioventricular block
AVD	aortic valve disease
AVR	aortic valve replacement
AVS	arteriovenous shunt
BBB	bundle branch block
BCLS	basic cardiac life support
BP	blood pressure
BPd, DBP	blood pressure – diastolic
bpm	beats per minute
BPs, SBP	blood pressure – systolic
CA	cardiac arrest, cancer, cardiac arrhythmia
CABG	coronary artery bypass graft
CABS	coronary artery bypass surgery
CAD	coronary artery disease
CEA	carotid endarterectomy
CHB	complete heart block

CHD	congenital heart disease, coronary heart disease
CHF	congestive heart failure
CO	cardiac output
CoA	coarctation of the aorta
CP	chest pain, cardiopulmonary
CPA	cardiopulmonary arrest, carotid phonoangiography
CPR	cardiopulmonary resuscitation
CV	cardiovascular
CVP	central venous pressure
CVS	cardiovascular system
DNR	do not resuscitate
DVT	deep vein thrombosis
ECC	emergency cardiac care, extracorporeal circulation
ECG, EKG	electrocardiogram
ECHO	echocardiography
EF	ejection fraction
EPS	electrophysiologic study
ETT	exercise tolerance test, exercise treadmill test
HBP	high blood pressure
HCM	hypertrophic cardiomyopathy
HCVD	hypertensive cardiovascular disease
HF	heart failure
HR	heart rate
HTN	hypertension
IABP	intra-aortic balloon pump
ICD	implantable cardiac defibrillator
ISH	isolated systolic hypertension
IV	intravenous, intraventricular
IVF	intravenous fluid, intravascular fluid
JVP	jugular venous pulse
LBBB	left bundle branch block

LBP	low blood pressure
LQTS	long QT syndrome
LVAD	left ventricular assist device
LVET	left ventricular ejection time
LVH	left ventricular hypertrophy
MI	myocardial infarction
MR	mitral regurgitation
MS	mitral stenosis
MVP	mitral valve prolapse
NSR	normal sinus rhythm
P	pulse
PAC	premature atrial contraction
PAD	peripheral arterial disease
PALS	pediatric advanced life support
PDA	patent ductus arteriosus
PEA	pulseless electrical activity
PPM	permanent pacemaker
PSVT, PST	paroxysmal supraventricular tachycardia
PTCA	percutaneous transluminal coronary angioplasty
PVC	premature ventricular contraction
PVD	peripheral vascular disease
RBBB	right bundle branch block
RHD	rheumatic heart disease
S_1, S_2	heart sound (first, second)
SBE	subacute bacterial endocarditis
SSS	sick sinus syndrome
SVT	supraventricular tachycardia
TET	treadmill exercise test
tPA, TPA	tissue plasminogen activator
TR	tricuspid regurgitation
TT	thrombolytic therapy
VF, Vfib, vent fib	ventricular fibrillation

VHD	valvular heart disease, ventricular heart disease
VPC	ventricular premature contraction
VSP	ventricular septal defect
VT, vtach	ventricular tachycardia
WPW	Wolff-Parkinson-White (syndrome)

NOTES

Sometimes an abbreviation can refer to two different things in the same system, and in another system.

Example:

ECC

Cardiovascular = emergency cardiac care **and** extracorporeal circulation

Female Reproductive = endocervical curettage

■ Endocrine System

AC	adrenal cortex
ACTH	adrenocorticotropic hormone
ADH	antidiuretic hormone
CAH	congenital adrenal hyperplasia
DI	diabetes insipidus
DKA	diabetic ketoacidosis
DM	diabetes mellitus
FSH	follicle-stimulating hormone
GH	growth hormone
HCG	human chorionic gonadotropin
HGF	human growth factor
ICSH	interstitial cell-stimulating hormone
IDDM	insulin-dependent diabetes mellitus

IGT	impaired glucose tolerance
JOD	juvenile-onset diabetes
LH	luteinizing hormone
MEA	multiple endocrine adenomatosis
MEN	multiple endocrine neoplasia
MSH	melanocyte-stimulating hormone
NIDDM	non-insulin-dependent diabetes mellitus
OXT	oxytocin
PRL	prolactin
PTH	parathyroid hormone
SIADH	syndrome of inappropriate ADH
STH	somatotropic hormone
T_3	triiodothyronine
T_4	thyroxine
TFT	thyroid function test
TSH	thyroid-stimulating hormone

■ Gastrointestinal System

abd	abdomen/abdominal
BE	barium enema
BM	bowel movement
BS	bowel sounds
CAH	chronic active hepatitis
CBD	common bile duct
CUC	chronic ulcerative colitis
D&V	diarrhea and vomiting
DU	duodenal ulcer
EGD	esophagogastroduodenoscopy
ERCP	endoscopic retrograde cholangiopancreatography
ESO, esoph	esophagus
GB	gallbladder

GBS	gallbladder series
GERD, GRD	gastroesophageal reflux disease
GI	gastrointestinal
HAV	hepatitis A virus
HBV	hepatitis B virus
HCl	hydrochloric acid
HCV	hepatitis C virus
HDV	hepatitis D virus
HI	hepatic insufficiency
IBD	inflammatory bowel disease
IBS	irritable bowel syndrome
IH	infectious hepatitis
IVC	intravenous cholangiography
LES	lower esophageal sphincter
LFT	liver function tests
LGI	lower gastrointestinal
LSK	liver, spleen and kidneys
NG, N-G	nasogastric (tube)
N/V	nausea and vomiting
OCG	oral cholecystogram
PEG	percutaneous endoscopic gastrostomy
PEM	protein-energy malnutrition
procto	proctoscopy
PU	peptic ulcer
PUD	peptic ulcer disease
RDA	recommended daily/dietary allowance
SBFT	small bowel follow-through
SBO	small bowel obstruction
SBS	small bowel series
TPN	total parenteral nutrition
UGI	upper gastrointestinal
VH	viral hepatitis

Integumentary System

BMK	birthmark
Bx	biopsy
decub	decubitus
DLE	discoid lupus erythematosus
DU	decubitus ulcer
EAHF	eczema, asthma, hay fever
EDR	electrodermal response
EGF	epidermal growth factor
HD	Hansen's disease (leprosy)
ID	intradermal
LE	lupus erythematosus
MM	malignant melanoma, multiple myeloma
PSS	progressive systemic sclerosis (scleroderma)
PUVA	psoralen ultraviolet A
SD	skin dose
SED	skin erythema dose
SG	skin graft
Ski, Sk	skin
SLE	systemic lupus erythematosus
SPF	skin protection factor
sq	squamous
SQ, SC, subcut, subq.	subcutaneous
STSG	split-thickness skin graft
TEN	toxic epidermal necrolysis
TSF	triceps skinfold
UV	ultraviolet
XP, XDP	xeroderma pigmentosum

■ Lymphatic & Immune Systems

Ab	antibody
ADC	AIDS-dementia complex
Ag	antigen, silver
AIDS	acquired immunodeficiency syndrome
ANA	antinuclear antibodies
APLS	antiphospholipid syndrome
ARC	AIDS-related complex
ARV	AIDS-related virus
EBV	Epstein-Barr virus
ELISA	enzyme-linked immunosorbent assay
GVHD	graft-versus-host disease
HD	Hodgkin's disease
HIV	human immunodeficiency virus
Ig	immunoglobulin
IM	infectious mononucleosis
IT	immunotherapy
KS	Kaposi sarcoma
LAK	lymphokine-activated killer (cells)
LE	lupus erythematosus
MAD	multiple autoimmune disorder
NHL	non-Hodgkin's lymphoma
NK	natural killer (cells)
OPV	oral poliovirus vaccine
PSS	progressive systemic sclerosis (scleroderma)
SCID	severe combined immunodeficiency disease
SLE	systemic lupus erythematosus
SS, Sjs	Sjögren syndrome
TAT	tetanus antitoxin
TLI	total lymphoid irradiation
vacc	vaccination

■ Muscular System

abd	abduction
ACL	anterior cruciate ligament
add	adduction
ADL	activities of daily living
ART	active resistance training
BMD	Becker muscular dystrophy
CTS	carpal tunnel syndrome
DMD	Duchenne muscular dystrophy
DTR	deep tendon reflex
EMG	electromyography
EMS	electric muscle stimulator
EOM	extraocular muscles
IM	intramuscular
Lig, L	ligament
M	muscle
MAMC	midarm muscle circumference
MD	muscular dystrophy
MG	myasthenia gravis
MH	malignant hyperthermia
mm	muscles
MN	myoneural
MS	musculoskeletal, muscle strength
musc	muscular, muscle
MVIC	maximum voluntary isometric contraction
NM	neuromuscular
PPMA	postpoliomyelitis muscular atrophy
PRE	progressive resistive exercise
RICE	rest, ice, compression, elevation
RSI	repetitive stress injuries

■ Nervous System

ACh	acetylcholine
AD	Alzheimer's disease, Alzheimer's dementia
ADD	attention deficit disorder
ADHD	attention deficit hyperactivity disorder
ALD	adrenoleukodystrophy
ALS	amyotrophic lateral sclerosis (Lou Gehrig's disease)
anesth, anes	anesthesia
ANS	autonomic nervous system
BAER	brainstem auditory evoked response
BBB	blood-brain barrier
BD	brain dead
BEAM	brain electrical activity mapping
CBF	cerebral blood flow
CJD	Creutzfeldt-Jakob disease (Mad Cow disease)
CNE	chronic nervous exhaustion
CNS	central nervous system
CP	cerebral palsy
CSF	cerebrospinal fluid
CVA	cerebrovascular accident
CVD	cerebrovascular disease
DAI	diffuse axonal injury
DT	delirium tremens
ECT	electroconvulsive therapy
EEG	electroencephalogram
EST	electric shock therapy
GAD	generalized anxiety disorder
GAS	general adaptation syndrome

HD	Huntington's disease
ICH	intracerebral hemorrhage
ICP	intracranial pressure
IQ	intelligence quotient
LMN	lower motor neuron
LOC	level/loss of consciousness
LP	lumbar puncture
MA	mental age
MBD	minimal brain dysfunction
MND	motor neuron disease
MS	multiple sclerosis
NCS	nerve conduction study
NF	neurofibromatosis
NGF	nerve growth factor
NTD	neural tube defect
OBS	organic brain syndrome
OCD	obsessive compulsive disorder
OMD	organic mental disorders
PD	Parkinson's disease, psychotic depression, psychotic dementia
PNI	peripheral nerve injury
PNS	peripheral nervous system
PTSD	posttraumatic stress disorder
RIND	reversible ischemic neurologic deficit
SAD	seasonal affective disorder
Sz	seizure
TBI	traumatic brain injury
TENS	transcutaneous electrical nerve stimulation
TGA	transient global amnesia
TIA	transient ischemic attack
UMN	upper motor neuron

■ Reproductive System – Female

Ab, AB	abortion
AFP	alpha fetoprotein
ARM, AROM	artificial rupture of membranes
ART	assisted reproductive technology
BSE	breast self-examination
BSO	bilateral salpingo-oöphorectomy
BWS	battered woman syndrome
C section, CS	Caesarean section
CVS	chorionic villus sampling
Cx	cervix
D&C	dilation and curettage
D&E	dilation and evacuation
DUB	dysfunctional uterine bleeding
ECC	endocervical curettage
EDC	estimated date of confinement
EDD	estimated date of delivery
EFM	electronic fetal monitor
ERT	estrogen replacement therapy
FHR	fetal heart rate
FHT	fetal heart tone
FTND	full-term normal delivery
GDM	gestational diabetes mellitus
GIFT	gamete intrafallopian transfer
grav	pregnancy
GYN	gynecology
HCG	human chorionic gonadotropin
HDN	hemolytic disease of the newborn
HRT	hormone replacement therapy
HSG	hysterosalpingography
IDM	infant of a diabetic mother
IUD	intrauterine device

IUFD	intrauterine fetal distress
IUP	intrauterine pregnancy
IVF	in vitro fertilization
L&D	labor and delivery
LDRP	labor, delivery, recovery, postpartum
LMP	last menstrual period
NB	newborn
ND	normal delivery
OB	obstetrics
OB/GYN	obstetrics and gynecology
OCP	oral contraceptive pills
Pap smear	Papanicolaou smear
para	number of viable births
PID	pelvic inflammatory disease
PIH	pregnancy induced hypertension
PMS	premenstrual syndrome
POU	placenta, ovary, uterus
SAB	spontaneous abortion
SVD	spontaneous vaginal delivery
TAb, TAB	therapeutic abortion
TAH	total abdominal hysterectomy
TOP	termination of pregnancy
TSS	toxic shock syndrome
UC	uterine contractions
VH	vaginal hysterectomy
ZIFT	zygote intrafallopian transfer

■ Reproductive System – Male

AIH	artificial insemination, homologous
BPH	benign prostatic hypertrophy
ED	erectile dysfunction
HSV	herpes simplex virus
NGU	non-gonococcal urethritis

NPT	nocturnal penile tumescence
PSA	prostate-specific antigen
RPR	rapid plasma reagin (test)
SPP	suprapubic prostatectomy
STD	sexually transmitted disease
TDF	testes determining factor
TFS	testicular feminization syndrome
TSE	testicular self-examination
TUR, TURP	transurethral resection of the prostate
VD	venereal disease
VDG	venereal disease – gonorrhea
VDS	venereal disease – syphilis

■ Respiratory System

ABC	airway, breathing and circulation
ABG	arterial blood gases
AR	artificial respiration
ARD	acute respiratory disease
ARDS	adult/acute respiratory distress syndrome
ARF	acute respiratory failure
BAC	bronchoalveolar cells
BAL	bronchoalveolar lavage
BPD	bronchopulmonary dysplasia
CF	cystic fibrosis
CNH	central neurogenic hyperventilation
CO_2	carbon dioxide
COLD	chronic obstructive lung disease
COPD	chronic obstructive pulmonary disease
CPAP	continuous positive airway pressure
CPE	chronic pulmonary emphysema

CPR	cardiopulmonary resuscitation
CPT	chest physiotherapy
CRD	chronic respiratory disease
CSR	Cheyne-Stokes respiration
CXR	chest x-ray
DOE	dyspnea on exertion
DPT	diphtheria, pertussis and tetanus
EIA	exercise-induced asthma
ERV	expiratory reserve volume
FEF	forced expiratory flow
FEV	forced expiratory volume
FRC	functional residual capacity
FVC	forced vital capacity
HBOT	hyperbaric oxygen therapy
HMD	hyaline membrane disease
IC	inspiratory capacity
IMV	intermittent mandatory ventilation
IPPB	intermittent positive pressure breathing
IRDS	infant respiratory distress syndrome
IRV	inspiratory reserve volume
LRI	lower respiratory infection
LTB	laryngotracheobronchitis
MBC	maximum breathing capacity
MV	minute volume
MVV	maximal voluntary ventilation
NSCLC	non-small cell lung cancer
O_2	oxygen
$PaCO_2$	partial pressure of arterial carbon dioxide
PaO_2	partial pressure of arterial oxygen
pCO_2	partial pressure of CO_2
PE	pulmonary embolism
PEEP	positive end expiratory pressure
PFT	pulmonary function test

PND	paroxysmal nocturnal dyspnea
pO_2	partial pressure of O_2
PPD	purified protein derivative (TB test)
PPH	primary pulmonary hypertension
PTX, Pnx, Px	pneumothorax
PuD, PD	pulmonary disease
R, resp	respiration
RD	respiratory disease
RDS	respiratory distress syndrome
RM	respiratory movement
RQ	respiratory quotient
RR	respiratory rate, regular respirations
RT	respiratory therapy
RV	residual volume
SCLC	small cell lung cancer
SIDS	sudden infant death syndrome
SOB	shortness of breath
T&A	tonsillectomy and adenoidectomy
TB	tuberculosis
TBT	tracheobronchial tree
TCDB	turn, cough and deep breathe
TLC	total lung capacity
TV	tidal volume
UAO	upper airway obstruction
URI	upper respiratory infection
VC	vital capacity
VO_2	oxygen consumption
V/Q	ventilation-perfusion ratio

■ Skeletal System

AEA	above elbow amputation
AFO	ankle-foot orthosis
AKA	above knee amputation
AROM	active range of motion

BEA	below elbow amputation
BKA	below knee amputation
BSF	basal skull fracture
C1-C7	cervical vertebrae
CDH	congenital dislocation of hip
CPM	continuous passive motion
DJD	degenerative joint disease
FRJM	full range of joint movement
FROM	full range of motion
Fx	fracture
HD	herniated disk
IVD	intervertebral disk
JRA	juvenile rheumatoid arthritis
jt, jnt	joint
KB	knee brace
Kj	knee jerk
L1-L5	lumbar vertebrae
LBP	low back pain
LOM	limitation of motion/movement, loss of motion/movement
LS	lumbosacral
OA	osteoarthritis
OAWO	opening abductory wedge osteotomy
OM	osteomalacia, osteomyelitis
ORIF	open reduction internal fixation
Ortho	orthopedics
PEMF	pulsing electromagnetic field
PKR	partial knee replacement
PROM	passive range of motion
RA	rheumatoid arthritis
RF	rheumatoid factor
ROM	range of motion
S1-S5	sacral vertebrae
sh, shld	shoulder

skel, sk	skeletal
T1-T12	thoracic vertebrae
THR	total hip replacement
TKA	total knee arthroplasty
TKR	total knee replacement
TMJ	temporomandibular joint
TX, Tx	traction

■ Special Senses: Ear

AC	air conduction
AD	right ear
AOM	acute otitis media
AS	left ear
AU	both ears
CAPD	central auditory processing disorder
dB	decibel
EE	eye and ear
ENT	ear, nose and throat
ET	eustachian tube
HD	hearing distance
HL	hearing level, hearing loss
OM	otitis media
ORL	otorhinolaryngology
SOM	serous otitis media
TM	tympanic membrane
VRA	visual reinforcement audiometry

■ Special Senses: Eye

acc	accommodation
ARMD	age-related macular degeneration
AS, Ast, Astigm	astigmatism
DV	distance vision
dv	double vision
E	eye

ECCE	extracapsular cataract extraction
EENT	eye, ear, nose and throat
EM	emmetropia
ENG	electronystagmography
EOM	extraocular movement
ERG	electroretinography
ET	esotropia
ICCE	intracapsular cataract extraction
IOL	intraocular lens
IOP	intraocular pressure
L&A	light and accommodation
L&D	light and distance
LE	left eye
M, My	myopia
NREM	non-rapid eye movement
NV	near vision
OD	right eye
OS	left eye
OU	each eye
PD	interpupillary distance
PERRLA	pupils equal, round, react to light and accommodation
RE	right eye
REM	rapid eye movement
RK	radial keratotomy
SMD	senile macular degeneration
VA	visual acuity
VF	visual field
XT	exotropia

■ Urinary System

AGN	acute glomerulonephritis
AHC	acute hemorrhagic cystitis
APD	adult polycystic disease
APORF	acute postoperative renal failure
ARF	acute renal failure

ATN	acute tubular necrosis
BUN	blood urea nitrogen
CAPD	continuous ambulatory peritoneal dialysis
cath.	catheter, catheterization
CRF	chronic renal failure
ESRD	end-stage renal disease
ESWL	extracorporal shockwave lithotripsy
GFR	glomerular filtration rate
GU	genitourinary
HD	hemodialysis
IC	interstitial cystitis
I&O	intake and output
IVC	intravenous cholangiography
IVP	intravenous pyelography
IVU	intravenous urography
KUB	kidney, ureter and bladder
NPN	non-protein nitrogen
NSU	non-specific urethritis
PD	peritoneal dialysis
PKD	polycystic kidney disease
PKU	phenylketonuria
RPF	renal plasma flow
RPG	retrograde pyelogram
RTA	renal tubular acidosis
RUG	retrograde urethrogram
TRBF	total renal blood flow
UA, U/A	urinalysis
UO, UOP	urinary output
Urol	urology
UTI	urinary tract infection
VCUG	voiding cystourethrogram

Glossary

A

a-, an-	without, not
ab-	away from
abdomin/o	abdomen
ablat/o	to remove, take away
abrad/o, abras/o	to scrape off
acanth/o	thorny, spiny
acar/o	mites
acid/o	acid, sour, bitter
acous/o	hearing
acoust/o	hearing, sound
acr/o	extremities
actin/o	ray, radiation
acu-	needle
acu/o, acut/o	sharp, severe
ad-	toward, near
aden/o	gland
adenoid/o	adenoids
adip/o	fat
adren/o	adrenal glands
aer/o	air, gas
agglutin/o	clumping
agit/o	rapidity, restlessness
-agogue	producer, leader
-agra	severe pain
alb/o, albin/o	white
albumin/o	albumin
alges/o, -algesia	pain sensitivity
-algia	pain
allo-	other, different
alveol/o	alveolus

ambi-	around, on both sides, about
ambly/o	dim, dull
ambul/o	to walk
ammon/o	ammonium
amni/o	amnion
amphi-	around, on both sides
amyl/o	starch
an/o	anus
ana-	up, backward, against
andr/o	male
aneurysm/o	aneurysm
angi/o	vessel
anis/o	unequal
ankyl/o	stiff, crooked, bent
anomal/o	irregular
ante-	before, forward
anter/o	front
anthrac/o	coal, carbon, carbuncle
anthrop/o	man, human being
anti-	against
antr/o	antrum
aort/o	aorta
-apheresis	separation, removal
aphth/o	ulcer
apic/o	apex
apo-	away, separation
aque/o	water
arachn/o	spider
arch/e, -arche, arch/i	first
arsenic/o	arsenic
arteri/o	artery
arteriol/o	arteriole
arthr/o	joint
articul/o	joint
aspir/o, aspirat/o	inhaling, removal
-assay	to examine, analyze
asthen/o, -asthenia	weakness

astr/o	star, star-shaped
atel/o	incomplete, imperfect
ather/o	fatty substance, plaque
atmo-	steam, vapor
-atresia	closure, occlusion
atreto-	closed, lacking an opening
atri/o	atrium
atto-	one-quintillionth (10^{-18})
audi/o, audit/o	hearing
aur/o, auricul/o	ear
auscult/o, auscultat/o	to listen
auto-	self
aux/o	growth, acceleration
axi/o	axis
axill/o	armpit
azot/o	nitrogen, urea

B

bacteri/o	bacteria
balan/o	glans penis
balne/o	bath
bar/o	weight, pressure
bary-	heavy, dull, hard
bas/o, basi/o	base, foundation
-basia	walking
batho-, bathy-	deep, depth
bi-	two
bibli/o	books
bil/i	bile
bi/o, bio-	life, living
blast/o, -blast	early embryonic stage, immature
blenn/o	mucus
blephar/o	eyelid
-boulia, -bulia	will

brachi/o	arm
brachy-	short
brady-	slow
brom/o	bromine-containing compound, odor
bronch/o	bronchus
bronchiol/o	bronchiole
bucc/o	cheek
burs/o	bursa

C

cac/o	bad, ill
calcane/o	heel
calci/o	calcium
calcul/o, -calculia	to compute
cali/o	calyx
calor/i	heat
campt/o	bent
capn/o, -capnia	carbon dioxide
caps/o, capsul/o	capsule, container
carb/o	carbon
carcin/o	cancer
cardi/o	heart
cari/o	caries, rottenness
carp/o	wrist
cata-	down, under
-cataphasia	affirmation
cathar/o, cathart/o	cleansing, purging
-cathisia, -kathisia	sitting
caud/o	tail
caus/o, cauter/o	burn, burning
cav/o, cavit/o	hollow, cavity

cec/o	cecum
-cele	hernia, swelling
celi/o	abdomen
-centesis	surgical puncture of a cavity
centi-	one-hundredth (10^{-2})
centr/o	center
cephal/o	head
cerebell/o	cerebellum
cerebr/o	cerebrum, brain
cervic/o	neck, cervix
-chalasia	relaxation
cheil/o, chil/o	lip
cheir/o, chir/o	hand
chem/o	chemical, chemistry
-chesia, -chezia	defecation
chlor/o	green
chol/e	gall, bile
choledoch/o	common bile duct
chondr/o	cartilage
chori/o	chorion
-chroia	skin coloration
chrom/o	color
chron/o	time, timing
chrys/o	gold
chyl/o	chyle
-cide	killing, agent that kills
cine-	movement
circum-	around
cirrh/o	orange-yellow
-clasia, -clasis, -clast	break
cleid/o	clavicle
clin/o	to slope, bend
-clysis	irrigation, washing
coagul/o	coagulation, clotting
-coccus	berry-shaped bacterium
coccyg/o	coccyx

cochle/o	cochlea
-coimesis	sleeping
col/o	colon
colp/o	vagina
com-, con-	with, together
-coma	deep sleep
coni/o	dust
conjunctiv/o	conjunctiva
consci/o	awareness, aware
constrict/o	narrowing, binding
contra-	against, opposite
contus/o	to bruise
cor/o	pupil
corne/o	cornea
coron/o	heart
corpor/o	body
cortic/o	cortex
cost/o	rib
cox/o	hip
crani/o	skull
-crasia	mixture (good or bad), temperament
cric/o	ring
crin/o	secrete, separate
-crit	separate
critic/o	crisis, dangerous
cry/o	cold
crypt/o	hidden, concealed
crystall/o	crystal, transparent
cubit/o	elbow, forearm
culd/o	cul-de-sac
cune/o	wedge, wedge-shaped
cupr/o	copper
-cusis	hearing
cutane/o	skin

cyan/o	blue
cycl/o	ciliary body, circular
-cyesis	pregnancy
cyst/o	bladder, cyst
cyt/o, -cyte	cell

D

dacry/o	tear
dactyl/o	digit (finger or toe)
deca-	ten (10^1)
deci-	one-tenth (10^{-1})
demi-	half
dem/o	people
dent/i	tooth
derm/o, dermat/o	skin
desicc/o	to dry
-desis	surgical fixation, fusion
desm/o	ligament
deuter/o	second, secondary
dextr/o	right
di-	two
dia-	through, throughout
didym/o	a twin, testis
-didymus	conjoined twin
dilat/o	to enlarge, expand
dipl/o	double
dips/o	thirst
dis-	apart, to separate
dist/o	distant
dolich/o	long
dolor/o	pain
dors/o	back
drom/o, -drome	running
duct/o	to lead

duoden/o	duodenum
dynam/o	power, strength
-dynia	pain
dys-	bad, difficult, painful

E

ec-, ecto-	outside, out
echin/o	spiny, prickly
echo-	reverberating sound
eco-	environment
-ectasia, -ectasis	dilation, expansion
-ectomy	surgical removal
ectr/o	congenital absence
-edema	swelling
ele/o	oil
electr/o	electricity
embol/o	embolus
embry/o	embryo
-emesis	vomiting
-emia	blood condition
emmetr/o	the correct measure, proportioned
-emphraxis	stoppage, obstruction
en-, endo-	inside, within
enanti/o	opposite, opposed
encephal/o	brain
enter/o	intestines (small intestines)
eosin/o	red, rosy, dawn
epi-	above, over, upon
epididym/o	epididymis
epiglott/o	epiglottis
episi/o	vulva
equi-	equality, equal
erethism/o	irritation

erg/o	work
erythem/o	flushed, redness
erythr/o	red
eschar/o	scab
eso-	within
esophag/o	esophagus
esthesi/o, -esthesia	sensation, feeling
eti/o	cause
eu-	good, normal, well
eury-	wide, broad
ex-	out, away from
exa-	quintillion (10^{18})
excit/o	to arouse
exo-	outside, outward
extra-	outside

F

faci/o	face
-facient	to cause, make happen
fasci/o	fascia
febr/i	fever
femor/o	femur
femto-	one-quadrillionth (10^{-15})
ferr/i, ferr/o	iron
fet/o	fetus
fibr/o	fiber, fibrous
fibul/o	fibula
fil/i, fil/o, filament/o	thread, threadlike
flav/o	yellow
flect/o, flex/o	bend
flu/o, flux/o	to flow
fluor/o	fluorine
follicul/o	small sac, follicle

fore-	before, in front
-form	specified shape, form
frig/o, frigid/o	cold
funct/o	performance
fung/i	fungus, mushroom
fusc/o	dark brown

G

galact/o	milk
galvano-	direct electric current
gam/o	marriage, sexual union
gamet/o	gamete
gangli/o, ganglion/o	ganglion
gastr/o	stomach
ge/o	earth, soil
gel/o	to freeze, congeal
gemell/o	twins
-gen, gen/o	producing, generating
-genesis	production, formation
-genic	produced by, forming
geni/o	chin
genit/o	reproduction
ger/o, geront/o	aged, old age
gest/o, gestat/o	to bear
-geusia	taste
giga-	billion (10^9)
gigant/o	huge
gingiv/o	gums
glauc/o	gray, bluish green
gli/o	glue, neuroglia
-globin	protein
glomerul/o	glomerulus
gloss/o	tongue
gluc/o	glucose, sugar

glyc/o	glucose, sugar
gnath/o	jaw
gnos/o	knowledge
gon/o	genitals, semen
gonad/o	gonads
goni/o	angle
-grade	step
-gram	written record
granul/o	granules
-graph	instrument for recording
graph/o	writing
-graphy	process of recording
gravid/o	pregnancy
-gravida	pregnant woman
gust/o, gustat/o	taste
gynec/o	woman, female
gyr/o	circle, spiral

H

haph/e	touch
hapl/o	simple, single
hect/o	hundred (10^2)
helc/o	ulcer
heli/o	sun
-helminth, helminth/o	worm
hemi-	half
hem/o, hemat/o	blood
hepat/o	liver
heredo-	heredity
hetero-	different, other
hex-, hexa-	six
-hexia	condition
hepta-	seven
hidr/o	sweat
hirsut/o	hairy

hirud/i, hirudin/i	leech
hist/o	tissue
holo-	entire, complete
homeo-	likeness, constant, sameness
homo-	same, similar
hormon/o	hormone
humer/o	humerus
hyal/o	resembling glass, glassy
hydr/o	water, hydrogen
hygr/o	moisture
hymen/o	hymen
hyper-	above, excessive, beyond
hypn/o	sleep
hypo-	under, deficient, below
hypothalam/o	hypothalamus
hypsi-	high
hyster/o	uterus

I

iatr/o	treatment, physician
ichthy/o	fish
-ician	specialist
icter/o	jaundice
ide/o	idea, mental images
idi/o	individual, distinct, unknown
ile/o	ileum
ili/o	ilium
immun/o	protection, immune
infra-	below, beneath
inguin/o	groin
inter-	between
intra-	within
iod/o	iodine
ion/o	ion
ipsi-	same

ir/o, irid/o	iris
isch/o	suppress, restrain
ischi/o	ischium
is/o	equal
-ist	specialist
ithy-	erect, straight
-itis	inflammation
ixod/i	ticks

J

jaund/o	yellow
jejun/o	jejunum
juxta-	near

K

kal/i	potassium
kary/o	nucleus
kel/o	tumor, fibrous growth
ken/o	empty
kerat/o	horny tissue, cornea
keraun/o	lightning
keton/o	ketones
kilo-	thousand (10^3)
kinesi/o, -kinesia, -kinetic	movement
klept/o	theft, stealing
koil/o	hollow, concave, depressed
kraur/o	dry
kym/o	waves
kyph/o	humpback

L

-labile	unstable, perishable
lacrim/o	tear, lacrimal duct
lact/o	milk
lal/o, -lalia	speech, babble
lamin/o	lamina
lampr/o	clear
lapar/o	abdomen, abdominal wall
laryng/o	larynx
later/o	side
laxat/o	to slacken, relax, loosen
lecith/o	yolk, ovum
-legia	reading
lei/o	smooth
-lemma	confining membrane
lepid/o	flakes, scales
lepr/o	leprosy
-lepsy	seizure
lept/o	slender, thin, delicate
letharg/o	drowsiness
leuk/o	white
levo-	left
-lexia	speech, word
lien/o	spleen
ligament/o	ligament
ligat/o	binding, tying
lim/o	hunger
lingu/o	tongue
lip/o	fat
-lipsis	omit, fail
-listhesis	slipping
lith/o	stone, calculus
lob/o	lobe
logad/o	whites of the eyes

log/o, -log/-logue	word, speech, thought
-logist	specialist
-logy	study of
loph/o	ridge
lord/o	curvature, bending
lox/o	oblique, slanting
-lucent	light-admitting
luc/i	light
lucid/o	clear
lumb/o	loin
lumin/o	light
lute/o	yellow
luxat/o	dislocate
ly/o	to dissolve, loosen
lymph/o	lymph
-lysis	dissolution, breakdown

M

-malacia	softening
mamm/o	breast
-mania	madness, obsessive preoccupation
-masesis	mastication, chewing
mast/o	breast
maxill/o	maxilla
medi/o	middle
mediastin/o	mediastinum
medic/o	to heal, healing
medull/o	medulla, marrow
mega-	million (10^6)
mega-, megalo-	large
-megaly	enlargement
mel/o	limb, limbs

melan/o	black
meli-, melit-	honey, sugar
men/o	menses, menstruation
mening/o	meninges, membranes
ment/o	mind
mer/o	part
meso-	middle
meta-	after, beyond, change
metall/o	metal
-meter	instrument for measuring
method/o	procedure, technique
metr/o	uterus
-metry	process of measuring
micro-	one-millionth (10^{-6}), small
mi/o	less, smaller
milli-	one-thousandth (10^{-3})
-mimesis	imitation, simulation
mis/o	hatred of, aversion
-mnesia	memory
mogi-	difficult
mono-	one
morph/o	shape, form
mort/o	death
-motor	movement, motion
muc/o	mucus
multi-	many, much
muscul/o	muscle
mutilat/o	to maim, disfigure
my/o, myos/o	muscle
myc/o	fungus
myel/o	bone marrow, spinal cord
myring/o	eardrum
myx/o	mucus

N

nano-	one-billionth (10^{-9})
narc/o	numbness, stupor
nas/o	nose
nat/o	birth
natr/o	sodium
necr/o	death
neo-	new
nephr/o	kidney
neur/o	nerve
neutr/o	neutral
nev/o	mole, birthmark
noci-	to cause harm, injury or pain
noct/i	night
nod/o	knot
-noia	mind, will
nom/o	custom, law
nomen-	name
noni-	nine
norm/o	normal, usual
nos/o	disease
not/o	the back
nucle/o	nucleus
nulli-	none
nutri/o, nutrit/o	to nourish
nyct/o	night

O

obstetr/o	midwife
octa-, octi-	eight
ocul/o	eye
odont/o	tooth
-oid	resembling
-ole	little, small
ole/o	oil
olfact/o	smell
olig/o	scanty, few, little
-oma	tumor, mass
om/o	shoulder
omphal/o	navel
onc/o	tumor, mass
onych/o	nail
o/ö	egg, ovum
oöphor/o	ovary
ophry/o	eyebrow
ophthalm/o	eye
-opia, -opsia	vision
opisth/o	backward, behind
op/o	juice, face
-opsy	to view
opt/o	eye, vision
or/o	mouth
orch/o, orchi/o, orchid/o	testis
-orexia	appetite
organ/o	organ
ornith/o	bird
orth/o	straight, normal, correct
osche/o	scrotum
oscill/o	to swing
-osis	condition, status, abnormal increase
osm/o, -osmia	sense of smell, odor, impulse

osphresi/o, -osphresia	sense of smell, odor
oste/o	bone
ot/o	ear
ov/i, ov/o	egg, ovum
ovari/o	ovary
ox/o, -oxia	oxygen
oxy-	sharp, quick, sour

P

pachy-	thick
-pagus	conjoined twins
palat/o	palate
pale/o	old
pali-, palin-	recurrence, repetition
palliat/o	to soothe, relieve
palp/o, palpat/o	to touch gently
palpebr/o	eyelid
palpit/o, palpitat/o	flutter, throbbing
pan-	all
pancreat/o	pancreas
pant/o	all, whole
papill/o	nipple-like, papilla
papul/o	papule, pimple
para-	alongside, near, beyond, abnormal
-para, -parous	to bear, bring forth
parasit/o	parasite
parathyroid/o	parathyroid gland
-paresis	partial paralysis
-partum	childbirth, labor
patell/o	patella
path/o	disease
-pause	cessation
pector/o	chest

ped/o	foot, child
pedicul/o	louse
pel/o	mud
pelv/i	pelvis
-penia	deficiency
pent-, penta-	five
-pepsia	digestion
per-	through, throughout
percuss/o	to tap
peri-	around, surrounding
perine/o	perineum
peritone/o	peritoneum
per/o	deformed, maimed
perone/o	fibula
perspir/o	breathe through
pest/i	plague, pests
peta-	quadrillion (10^{15})
-petal	moving toward, seeking
petr/o	stone, petrous region of temporal bone
-pexy	fixation
phac/o	lens
phag/o, -phagia	eating, ingestion
phak/o	lens
phalang/o	phalanges
phall/o	penis
phaner/o	visible, apparent
pharmac/o	drugs
phas/o, -phasia	speech
phe/o	dusky
phen/o	appearance
-pheresis	removal
-phil, -philia	affinity for, tendency toward
phim/o	muzzle
phleb/o	vein

phob/o, -phobia	fear, aversion
phon/o, -phonia	voice, sound
phor/o, -phore	bearer, processor
-phoresis	bearing, transmission
phosphat/o	phosphate
phot/o	light
phren/o	mind, diaphragm
phyc/o	seaweed, algae
phyl/o	race, species, type
-phylaxis	protection
phyll/o	leaf, leaf-like
-phyma	tumor, growth
phys/o	air, gas
physi/o	nature
physic/o	physical, natural
-physis	growth, growing
phyt/o, -phyte	plant
pico-	one-trillionth (10^{-12})
picr/o	bitter
pies/i, -piesis, piez/o	pressure
pil/o	hair
pimel/o	fat, fatty
pin/o	to drink
pineal/o	pineal gland
pituitar/o	pituitary gland
plagi/o	slanting, oblique
plan/o	flat, level, wandering
plant/o	sole of the foot
-plasm	formation, growth
plasm/o	plasma, formative substance
-plasty	surgical correction/repair
platy-	broad, flat
ple/o	more
-plegia	paralysis
plesi/o	nearness, similarity

pless/i	striking
pleur/o	pleura
plex/o	network (nerves or vessels), plexus
plic/o, plicat/o	to fold, pleat
-ploid, -ploidy	number of chromosome sets
pluri-	more, several
-pnea	breath, breathing
pneum/o	lung, air
pneumon/o	lung, air
pod/o	foot
-poiesis	formation
poikil/o	variation, irregular
poli/o	gray (matter)
poly-	many, much
pon/o	fatigue, overwork, pain
por/o, -pore	opening, passageway
-porosis	porous, decrease in density
-posia	drinking
posit/o	arrangement, place
post-	after, behind
poster/o	behind, toward the back
potenti/o	power, strength
-prandial	meal
-praxia	action, activity
pre-	before, in front of
presby-	aging, elderly
primi-	first
-privia	loss, deprivation
pro-	before
proct/o	rectum, anus
pros/o	forward, anterior
prosop/o	face
prostat/o	prostate gland

prot/o	first
prote/o	protein
proxim/o	near
prurit/o	itching
psamm/o	sand, sand-like material
pselaphes/o	touch
pseudo-	false
psor/o	itching
psych/o	mind
psychr/o	cold
-pterygium	abnormality of the conjunctiva
pteryg/o	wing-shaped
-ptosis	prolapse, drooping
ptyal/o	saliva
-ptysis	spitting
pub/o	pubis
pulmon/o	lung
puls/o, pulsat/o	to beat, beating
-puncture	to pierce a surface
pupill/o	pupil
purgat/o	cleansing
purpur/i	purple
purul/o	pus formation
py/o	pus
pycn/o, pykn/o	thick, dense
pyel/o	renal pelvis
pyg/o	buttocks
pyl/e	portal vein
pylor/o	pylorus
pyr/o	heat, fever, fire
pyret/o	fever
pyrex/o	feverishness, fever

Q

quadri-	four
quinque-	five
quint/i	fifth

R

rachi/o	spine
radi/o	x-ray, radiation
radicul/o	nerve root
ram/i	branch
re-	back, again
-receptor, -ceptor	receiver
rect/o	rectum
reflex/o, reflect/o	to bend back
registrat/o	recording
relaps/o	to slide back
ren/o	kidney
respir/o, respirat/o	breath, breathing
resuscit/o	to revive
reticul/o	net-like
retin/o	retina
retract/o	drawing back
retro-	behind, backward
rhabd/o	rod
rhabdomy/o	striated/skeletal muscle
rhe/o	flow, current, stream
rhin/o	nose
rhiz/o	root
rhod/o	red, rosy
rhytid/o	wrinkle
rose/o	rosy
rot/o, rotat/o	turn, revolve

-rrhage, -rrhagia	excessive flow, profuse fluid discharge
-rrhaphy	suture
-rrhea	flow, discharge
-rrhexis	rupture
-rrhythm/o	rhythm
rubr/i, rubr/o	red

S

sacchar/o	sugar
sacr/o	sacrum
salping/o	fallopian tube
sangu/i, sanguin/o	blood
sanit/a	health
sap/o	soap
sapr/o	rotten, decay
sarc/o	flesh
saur/o	lizard
scaph/o	a scapha, boat-shaped
scapul/o	scapula
scat/o	feces
scel/o, -scelia	leg
-schisis, schist/o	split, cleft
schiz/o	split, division
scint/i	spark
scirrh/o	hard
scler/o	sclera
-sclerosis	hardening
scolec/o	worm
scoli/o	crooked, twisted
-scope	instrument for visual examination
-scopy	visual examination
scot/o	darkness

scrib/o, script/o	to write
seb/o	sebum
-sect	to cut
secund/i	second
sedat/o	to calm
semi-	half
semin/i	semen
senil/o	old, old age
sens/o, sensat/o	feeling, perception
sensor/i	sensory
-sepsis, septic/o	putrefaction, putrefying
sept/o	partition
sept-, septi-	seven
ser/o	serum, serous
sesqui-	one and a half
sex-	six
sial/o	saliva
sicc/o	to dry
sider/o	iron
sigmoid/o	sigmoid colon
silic/o	silica, quartz
sinistr/o	left
sin/o, sinus/o	cavity, sinus
sit/o	food
skelet/o	skeleton
soci/o	social, society
sodi/o	compound containing sodium
solut/o	dissolved
somat/o	body
-some	body
somn/i, -somnia	sleep
son/o	sound
span/o	scanty, scarce
-spasm, spasm/o	involuntary contraction
spectr/o	image, spectrum

sperm/o, spermat/o	spermatozoa
sphen/o	wedge, sphenoid bone
spher/o	round, sphere
sphygm/o	pulse
-sphyxia	pulse
spin/o	spinal cord, spine
spir/o	breath, breathing
splanchn/o	viscera
splen/o	spleen
spondyl/o	vertebrae, spinal column
spongi/o	spongelike, spongy
spor/o	spore, seed
squam/o	squamous, scales
-stabile	stable, fixed
-stalsis	contraction
staped/o	stapes
staphyl/o	uvula, grape-like clusters
-stasis	standing still, standing
-stat	device/instrument for keeping something stationary
steat/o	fat
sten/o, -stenosis	narrowed, constricted
stere/o	solid, three-dimensional
steril/o	barren
stern/o	sternum
steth/o	chest
sthen/o, -sthenia	strength
stich/o, -stichia	rows
stigmat/o	mark, point
stomat/o	mouth
-stomy	surgical opening
strat/i	layer

strept/o	twisted, curved
strict/o	to tighten, bind
-stroma	supporting tissue of an organ
stroph/o	twisted
sub-	under, beneath
succ/o	juice
suct/o	to suck
sud/o	sweat
sulc/o	furrow, groove
super-	above, beyond
supra-	above, beyond
suspend/o, suspens/o	to hang up, suspend
sym-, syn-	with, together
symptom/o	occurrence
synaps/o, synapt/o	point of contact, to join
syndesm/o	ligament, connective tissue
synov/o	synovia, synovial membrane
syphil/o	syphilis
syring/o	tube, fistula
system/o	system
systol/o	contraction
syzygi/o	bound together, conjunction

T

tachy-	fast
tact/o	touch
tal/o	talus
taph/o	grave
tapin/o	low
tars/o	tarsus, edge of eyelid
tauto-	identical, same
tax/o, -taxia	coordination
techn/o	skill, art

tect/o	rooflike
tegment/o	covering
tel/e	end, distant
tel/o	end
tele/o	perfect, complete
temp/o, tempor/o	period of time, the temples
ten/o	tendon
tenont/o	tendon
tens/o, -tension	stretched, strained
tephr/o	gray (ashen)
tera-	trillion (10^{12})
terat/o	monster
termin/o	boundary, limit
terti-	third
test/o, testicul/o	testis
tetan/o	tetanus
tetra-	four
thalam/o	thalamus
thanat/o	death
thec/o	sheath
thel/o	nipple
theor/o	speculation
therapeut/o, -therapy	treatment
theri/o	animals
therm/o	heat
thigm/o	touch
thio-	presence of sulfur
thorac/o	chest
thromb/o	clot, thrombus
-thymia	mind, emotions
thym/o	thymus gland
thyr/o	thyroid gland
tibi/o	tibia
toc/o, -tocia	childbirth, labor
-tome	instrument for cutting
tom/o	a cutting (section/layer)

-tomy	surgical incision
ton/o	tone, tension
tonsill/o	tonsils
top/o	particular place or area
torpid/o	sluggish, inactive
tors/o	twisting, twisted
tox/o, toxic/o	poison
trache/o	trachea
trachel/o	neck
trachy-	rough
trans-	across
traumat/o	trauma, injury, wound
trem/o, tremul/o	shaking, trembling
-tresia	opening, perforation
tri-	three
tri/o	to sort out, sorting
trich/o	hair
-tripsy	to crush, break
troph/o, -trophy	nourishment, growth
-tropia	to turn
tub/o	tube
tubercul/o	tubercle, tuberculosis
tumesc/o, -tumescence	swelling
turbid-	cloudy, confused
turg/o, turgid/o	to swell, swollen
tympan/o	eardrum (tympanic membrane)
typ/o, -type	class, representative form
typhl/o	cecum, blindness
typh/o	typhus, typhoid
tyr/o	cheese, caseous

U

-ule	little, small
ul/o	scar, scarring
ultra-	beyond, excess
un-	not, reversal
ungu/o	nail
uni-	one
uran/o	palate
-uresis	urination
ureter/o	ureter
urethr/o	urethra
-uria	urine condition
uric/o	uric acid
urin/o	urine
ur/o	urine
uter/o	uterus
uve/o	uvea
uvul/o	uvula

V

vaccin/o	vaccine
vag/o	vagus nerve
vagin/o	vagina
valv/o, valvul/o	valve
vari/o, variat/o	change, vary
varic/o	varicose veins
vas/o	vessel, vas deferens
vascul/o	blood vessel
ven/o	vein
venere/o	sexual intercourse
ventil/o	to aerate, oxygenate
ventr/o	belly, front of the body

ventricul/o	ventricle of the heart or brain
venul/o	venule
verm/i	worm
verruc/i	wart
vers/o, -verse	turn, turning
vertebr/o	vertebra
vesic/o	urinary bladder
vesicul/o	seminal vesicle, a vesicle
vestibul/o	vestibule
vibr/o, vibrat/o	to quiver, shake
vir/o	virus
viril/o	masculine, manly
viscer/o	internal organs
viscid/o, viscos/o	sticky, glutinous
vitell/o	yolk
vit/o, vital/o	life
vitre/o	glassy, vitreous body
viv/i	life, alive
-volemia	blood volume
volut/o, volv/o	to roll
vulv/o	vulva

X

xanth/o	yellow
xen/o	strange, foreign matter
xer/o	dry
xiph/o	sword-shaped, xiphoid

Z

zon/i, zon/o	zone, encircling region
zo/ö	animal
zyg/o	union, junction
zym/o	enzyme, ferment